Treatment for Youth with Sexual Behavior Problems

A practical guide for identifying treatment programs
that empower clients and transform lives

Shanti Duncan, Ph.D.

The events and conversations in this book have been set down to the best of the author's ability, although names and details have been changed to protect the privacy of individuals. The information given in this book should not be treated as a substitute for professional medical advice; always consult a medical practitioner. Any use of information in this book is at the reader's discretion and risk. Neither the author nor the publisher can be held responsible for any loss, claim, or damage arising out of the use, or misuse, of the suggestions made, the failure to take medical advice, or for any material on third-party websites.

First Printing:

ISBN: 979-8-9878686-0-7

Contact author:

Shanti Duncan

12407 North Mopac Expwy Ste.250-285

Austin TX 78758-2475

shanti.duncan.lpc@gmail.com

What Others Are Saying

"Talking about "sex offenders" and even "juvenile sex offenders," as we for so many years labeled people who sexually offended, was a conversation held mostly among professionals in the field. Dr. Duncan's book, Treatment for Youth with Sexual Behavior Problems, is a game changer! Her book is a conversation that she is having with common folk, everyday people, families, parents, loved ones, and even the person who sexually offended. Notwithstanding the ordinary language she uses, her knowledge and experience in the field are evident from beginning to end, as are her wisdom, compassionate worldview, and treatment style. For anyone, be it a professional in the field or someone seeking to understand the offending behavior of a loved one, this book provides solid, common-sense information. Commendably, there is no psychobabble here. Dr. Duncan describes, in plain English, the concepts, the process, and the experience of not only treating persons who sexually offend but also loving them."

~ Nicolas Carrasco, Psychologist, LSOTP, Author of Beacon - Treatment Manual for Juveniles with Sexual Behavior Problems

"The topic of sexual behavior problems has rarely been written about in a skillful, highly readable fashion and with the level of clarity and insight of this innovative book. This a valuable resource, for both novice and veteran clinicians, of what can be effective in good quality treatment of youth with said issues."

~ Dr. Monica Gomez, Psy.D., LSOTP

"I have worked with Shanti Duncan and other sex offense-specific treatment providers for over twenty years. This book is an excellent resource for information about treatment for youth and for people who want to understand the role polygraph exams play in treatment."

~ **Sabino Martinez, Certified Polygraph Examiner**

"As probation officers, our main role is to monitor probation conditions and enforce violations to ensure community safety. As much as we wish it were, it is not simple. It is important to see past the violation and understand the "why" behind the behaviors. I have been lucky to work very closely with Dr. Duncan to help many youth and families make it through this journey and move on to become successful adults. I've seen firsthand how compassion and respect will lead to success over antiquated shame-based methods. Learning to understand the therapeutic process requires those working with youth in sexual behavior treatment programs to be open-minded and work collaboratively with LSOTPs to formulate recommendations and plans that are not only in the child's best interest but will ensure community safety. Dr. Duncan does a phenomenal job of walking you through the entire process and will help you to understand the reasoning behind each stage of treatment. Whether you are new to the field or a twenty-year veteran, this book will no doubt be a beneficial aid to guide you through your career in working with juveniles with sexual behavior problems."

~ **Lorena Moreno, Juvenile Probation Officer**

"Congratulations to Dr. Duncan! Her book Treatment for Youth with Sexual Behavior Problems is an excellent resource for treatment providers. She combines an easy read with evidence-based information and practices that help professionals better understand work with youth with sexual behavior problems. Her examples of cases are presented in a narrative as lessons learned and reflections rather than dry and complicated clinical facts. Her sensitivity and passion are evident in her writing, and she makes poignant points for us to pause and reflect on our own biases in working with youth. She helps us to increase our awareness of diversity in this population and reminds us that we are working with children who are not yet developed cognitively, sexually, or emotionally. What a great tool to have with this guide!"

~ **Diana Garza-Louis, LPC-S, LMFT-S, RPT-S**

Table of Contents

Introduction

A surefire way to make small talk with strangers even more awkward than usual is to answer the question "What do you do?" with "I am a therapist who works mostly with people who have experienced trauma and with people with sexual behavior problems." There are a lot of wonderful reasons to work in this field. The length of time that clients spend in treatment gives them a chance to form deep rich therapeutic relationships. Often, there is an opportunity to interrupt long-standing multigenerational patterns of abuse and dysfunction. There is the opportunity to help heal existing trauma and prevent future trauma before it happens. It is very rewarding to see the changes that people and families are able to make over time. Awkward small talk, especially for an introvert like me who is not good at or fond of small talk anyway, can be an amusing side effect.

The term "sex offender" has a lot of stigmas, and the idea of spending time around sex offenders can be scary or off-putting for people. As a whole, the treatment community is moving away from that term, and instead, we talk about people who have a sexual behavior problem or have committed a sex crime. The idea of working with people who have committed a sex offense can seem baffling or impossible to many individuals. When I started working with people who had committed sex crimes, I wondered what I had gotten myself into, but more striking was how people who knew me reacted. Mostly, they were equally worried about my well-being and fairly convinced I was crazy. My mom sent me a canister of mace and asked me to keep it with me, even though I told her I was not particularly worried about my safety. Even now, sometimes people will ask if I go to work armed. For many years I worked with a group of adult offenders in a more rural area of Texas. Some of the clients wondered why I would work with them without a gun. Some of that might be a side effect of living in Texas, where people assume that others might be armed. If you are wondering, the answer to that question is no, I do not go to work armed, and I have also never felt obligated to have the mace with me either, though I used to keep it in my work bag to make my mom feel better. I have been working in an outpatient setting with adults and adolescents who have gotten into legal trouble for their sexual behavior for over twenty years, and so far, I have never felt in danger.

Society has always had difficulty dealing with people who engage in inappropriate sexual behavior. The term "sex offender" generally provokes a lot of emotion, angst, and strong responses. Feelings about individuals who have committed a sex crime are typically more negative than those who have committed other types of crimes (Harper and Hicks, 2022). In part because of the stigma associated with the term "sex offender" and in part to acknowledge that when working with youth, we do not want to put big labels on children who are still developing, growing, and changing, I will generally be referring to my adolescent clients as "youth or juveniles with sexual behavior problems." It is a longer phrase than just saying "sex offenders," but it is more accurate. I was recently reminded of the importance of how things are worded when I was talking to a small group of therapists in a class where we talked about book writing. We were discussing the topics of the book we were each working on, and I stated that I was working on writing a book about working with juvenile sex offenders.

One person immediately said that "those people" should be executed; another said they should be tortured first. I do not know either of those people, but they are professional therapists. They changed the subject after I commented that not only would that involve killing many people, but since I was talking about juveniles, that would involve torturing and killing children. I didn't think that was a good way to treat people. After that conversation, I wondered if I would have gotten a different response if I had said I was working on a book for youth with sexual behavior problems. It has taken me some time to write this book, and I have taken a few versions of the same class, and each time I am asked about the topic of my book, I now answer by saying that I am writing about what works in treatment for youth with sexual behavior problems. Since I started using that phrasing, no one has suggested killing my clients. Most people are very positive about the importance of that kind of work—a very different response than I got before. I was not as careful with my language as I should have been that first time, partly because I knew I was talking to other therapists, so the shorthand seemed appropriate. It was a good reminder that words matter. Many people, even those in the mental health community, are not always willing to acknowledge people's capacity for change, especially when they find their behavior personally uncomfortable.

I am often asked if I think treatment works. It always makes me wonder why someone would think I would have spent my career doing something if I thought that it did not have any impact. The myth that people who commit sex crimes cannot be helped and will never change is persistent and problematic. It is, however, a myth; of course, not every client will benefit from treatment, but the vast majority of clients do, and the recidivism rate for juveniles who commit sex crimes is quite low. One study found that the rate of sexual reoffending in juveniles is about 5 percent for five years (Caldwell, 2016). Other studies find lower rates, and some find slightly higher rates. But overall, the rate of sexual reoffense for adolescents in legal trouble for their sexual behavior is very low. This is information that everyone working with these youth should know, and there is no reason to treat them as if they are irreparably damaged people destined for a life of crime.

People have, for good reason, strong feelings about how people who commit sex offenses should be treated and often have strong feelings about what they think will work or not work in the treatment and management of offenders. Unfortunately, even the strongest convictions about a topic do not mean that the person with strong feelings knows what they are talking about or that their ideas are supported by research. Most people's ideas of what sex offenders are like come from television shows, movies, and other media and are generally not particularly accurate.

Many years ago, I was visiting some relatives, and I was introduced to one of their neighbors, who was aware from the conversation that I was a treatment provider for people who had committed sex crimes. This man told me that he knew that women did not commit sex crimes, that it was only a thing that men did. I explained that that was not accurate information and that there were court-ordered girls and women on my caseload at that moment in time. Men and boys commit the majority of sex crimes; about 5 percent of adults who engage in illegal sexual behavior and 7 percent of adolescents who are under court supervision for a sex crime are female. My relatives' neighbor told me that was not true, that women do not think of sex like that, and therefore there were no women who commit sex crimes. He was totally convinced and remained convinced even after I was clear that, as someone who worked with women and girls who have committed sex crimes, I knew for sure that they existed. I even told him I had given presentations at conferences about working with girls with sexual behavior problems. My knowledge of the situation made no difference to his conviction that what he "knew" about women and sex crimes was true. It was an odd conversation. I thought for a minute about arguing that there was no such thing as condos or townhouses (he was a real estate agent) but decided that he probably would not have gotten my point. There was not any real reason to continue the conversation. My relatives have long since moved, and I did not have any other interactions with him, but it was a good reminder of how firmly people can believe in information they are convinced is true, even with evidence to the contrary. That is particularly true when the topic is something that people have a strong emotional reaction to. I have no idea why it was important for that man to believe that women were incapable of committing sex crimes, but clearly, that was a firmly held though inaccurate belief for him.

When I started working as a therapist, I was lucky enough to work with wonderful mentors and supervisors who helped me figure out what works and what my style is as a therapist. I was also lucky enough to start working with this population after the therapeutic community had figured out that shame-based treatment was ineffective and that treating juveniles as if they were just small adults was also ineffective. The people I was working with, and for the most part still work with, paid attention to the latest research and used the information they learned at conferences and training to make changes in their treatment program so it could be as effective as possible. None of them engaged in treatment modalities that treated clients as if they deserved to be treated badly. Not everyone has that opportunity, and I regularly run into therapists, probation officers, and other professionals who either do not have any colleagues in the field or who have found themselves working in programs that still use an old-style approach that has long been proven to be problematic, ineffective, and harmful. Treatment providers, probation officers, judges, district attorneys, and other professionals involved in decision-making about children in the justice system have too important a role to play to not be sure they are utilizing the best practices. All people, especially children, deserve to be treated with dignity and respect and be given the opportunity to change and grow and find their way to being happy, healthy, functioning members of society.

Finding a way to work effectively with clients while staying true to myself and how I approach therapeutic relationships was very useful and was not necessarily something that happened overnight. I wrote this book intending to lay out what we know at the moment about what is effective in working with youth who have committed a sex crime and to help people who work with children with sexual behavior problems be able to find their own voice and style to help them be the most effective and impactful they can be. This is a field that, while no longer in its infancy, is still relatively young, and the body of research we have to draw on is expanding rapidly. Professionals in the field must be willing to adjust to new information about treatment, risk assessment, and the best ways to help our clients find their way to healthy, well-adjusted lives.

People often ask me why I do the kind of work that I do. There are many ways to answer that question. One answer is that I like a challenge and am not fond of boredom. Working with clients who were court-ordered due to their sexual behavior is never dull. It is also very rewarding to help people make significant changes in their lives and be successful, healthy, safe, and functioning members of society. Working with people who have committed sex crimes is also about prevention. While it is a stereotype that every person who commits a sex crime has multiple victims, some of the people we work with have victimized more than one person. Working with individuals who commit sex crimes can protect other people they come into contact with in the future and sometimes is a key part in disrupting patterns of multi-generational abuse and trauma that have been happening in families for decades. No one person can fix the entirety of a problem, and my work will not stop sex crimes from happening, but many people working together can make a difference. There are many things we can each do that together will have a significant impact. That work can go a long way both in the pursuit of repairing the trauma of sexual violence and in the work of preventing future sexual violence from occurring in the first place.

Like most licensed professionals, I need to attend a certain number of continuing education units in my field regularly, so I attend and sometimes present at conferences about working with people who engage in inappropriate sexual behavior. I have noticed over the years that people, especially those who are newer in the field, are looking for a reliable source of information to know how to recognize good quality treatment and management programs. The idea for this book came from conversations I have had with people at conferences; therapists, probation officers, lawyers, judges, and other professional discussions. I hope that it will be an accessible, useful way to help people who work in this field and those who need to know more about this field feel more confident about their ability to work with this rewarding and challenging population. Perhaps it will also give you some good ways to make small talk more awkward if you are into that!

Chapter 1

History of Treatment Approaches

Over the last several decades, what we know about treating and managing adults and youth with sexual behavior problems has increased dramatically. Much of that information is in research journals which are not always accessible or of interest to the general public. Even professionals in this field often do not have access to research journals unless they also happen to teach at a university. It is important for the knowledge gained from research to not just sit on a shelf in a university library or behind a paywall online but be able to be practically used in clinical settings. My intention is for this book to serve as a way to get some of that information, both from research and clinical experience, to the professionals who work with these youth so that they and their clients can benefit from it.

In the beginning, all our information about working with people with sexual behavior problems came from a limited amount of research done with incarcerated adult offenders, mostly rapists and pedophiles. That group of people was not representative even of most adult offenders, let alone juveniles who engage in illegal sexual behavior. Today we have access to much broader sources of information, and the body of research continues to grow. There is more diversity in the types of populations we have information about. Not just adult incarcerated offenders but also outpatient clients and those who have committed a wide range of sex crimes. We have research from a more diverse group of researchers as well. We can now talk about the differences in various groups and categories of offenders and types of crimes. Not lumping everyone together has made an enormous difference in getting the correct type of treatment matched to the right clients. A growing body of research is specifically about working with juveniles, and there is also a growing body of research specifically about working with girls and women. As with most topics, the more we know and the less we generalize, the better we can be effective and useful to our clients and the larger community. There are still a lot of myths out there, both among the general population and—more damagingly—among mental health professionals, law enforcement professionals, and lawyers and judges. It is important that people stay in touch with what is new in the field, as what we "know" changes over time as we acquire more and better information. When learning about research and statistics in school, I can remember learning the phrase "garbage in, garbage out." We will inevitably get bad results if we make decisions based on bad data and faulty assumptions.

I have occasionally had people say that I am too soft-hearted or not hard enough on court-ordered clients when I talk about the problems with shame-based treatment or with aspects of the registration laws. Some people feel strongly that individuals who commit sex crimes deserve to be shamed and treated badly. I try to explain that it is not necessarily about being "nice" to clients for the sake of being nice. It is about the end goal. If we want people to be healthy, safe, functioning members of society, we need to do the things that will get them there. There is ample evidence that isolating, shaming, and humiliating people will only increase the risk of them continuing to act in problematic ways and being less likely to talk about that behavior with their treatment team. As a society and as a treatment and law enforcement community, we have to decide if the goal is simply to punish or if the goal is to hold people responsible for their behavior while also helping them make changes for the future. If you have read this far into the book, you already know by now which side of that question I come down on. Punishment just for punishment's sake does not help anyone, not the person who committed the crime, not the person who was victimized, and not the community either.

When people who had committed sex offenses were first sent to treatment, treatment providers often focused almost entirely on deviance and risk. It was thought that "Once a sex offender, always a sex offender," and providers would often use shame-based techniques with the idea of breaking someone down in order to build them up again. Clients were told they were deviant, would always be deviant, and needed to spend their lives away from others to ensure the community's safety. Of course, that turns out to not only be not true but also very damaging. We have lots of research and common sense that show us that treating people poorly, as if they are not really human and do not deserve dignity and respect, does not teach them to treat others with dignity and respect. We cannot teach people to treat others well and respect their boundaries while shaming them and conveying the message that there is no hope for them. That does not mean, by the way, that there are no consequences for behavior. It just means we can hold people accountable and expect them to take responsibility for their behavior without demeaning and dehumanizing them.

No one book can contain all the information there is to know on any subject, and this one is definitely no exception. It will provide a (relatively) brief overview of working with youth with sexual behavior problems and the components that make up good quality treatment programs. I hope this book will be helpful not only to treatment providers but also to the other professionals who work with youth with sexual behavior problems. Good quality treatment is a team effort that includes judges, lawyers, probation/parole officers, facility staff, parents, wraparound and support services, and the broader community. The more people who know what works, the more able we are to help these children get back on track to have fabulous futures. While reading this book, please also remember that while we have access to a much higher quality and a broader range of research than we did just a decade ago, this is still a field in development. The research gets better every day, and I would imagine in a decade, we will look and wonder why we did not see now what seems obvious to people in the future. As our field moves forward, I have no doubt that some of what is in this book will need updating and changing. It is important to keep in touch with growth and change in the field and to be able to evaluate the quality of the information you have and the new information as it emerges.

So let us start with some history because it is hard to know where you are going if you do not know where you have been. People who have gotten in trouble legally for their sexual behavior are pretty routinely ordered to sex offense-specific treatment, but the formal treatment of sex offenders is actually a relatively new field. The Association for the Treatment of Sexual Abusers (ATSA), the field's major professional organization, was formed in the 1980s. While ATSA is now an international organization, the story is that it started with a group of treatment providers and other professionals working in the field getting together for monthly lunch meetings to talk about their work. This group established the first practice standards for treating and evaluating people who had committed sex offenses. They eventually formed an official organization (at that time called the Association for the Behavioral Treatment of Sexual Aggressives) and created a code of ethics for treatment providers.

The name has undergone a couple of changes, from the Association for the Behavioral Treatment of Sexual Aggressives to the Association for the Behavioral Treatment of Sexual Abusers, and then finally to the current Association for the Treatment of Sexual Abusers (ATSA). Now and then, ATSA members discuss changing the name again as the current practice has gotten more comprehensive, and there is a lot more focus on prevention. As of when I am writing this, there is a vote happening about changing the name. Depending on the results of that vote, the acronym ATSA will still be used, but the full name may change to the Association for the Treatment and Prevention of Sexual Abuse.

As mentioned above, ATSA is now an international organization focusing on both treatment and research. The organization produces practice guidelines, ethical codes, and a peer-reviewed journal. In addition, ATSA hosts a large annual conference in various places across the US and Canada. Most recently, due to the current pandemic crisis, the conference was moved to an online format. There are also continuing education classes available for purchase through the ATSA website. As of this writing, ATSA has more than 3,000 members from more than twenty countries. These members include treatment providers, researchers, law enforcement, court and correction officers, victim advocates, and students. Many states have their own chapters, some of which also host regular conferences.

In addition to their annual conference, which is a great place to learn about what is going on in the field, ATSA also has a peer-reviewed journal, *Sexual Abuse*, another good resource for the latest research useful for those working in this field. The organization also publishes practice guidelines for working with adults, working with adolescents, a professional code of ethics, and many other reports on various topics accessible on their website.

The National Adolescent Perpetration Network (NAPN) was founded in 1983 to focus on the needs and requirements of youth with sexual behavior problems. This organization focused on distributing information about developmentally appropriate evidence-based treatment and assessing adolescents with sexual behavior problems. They did this primarily through annual conferences. A few years ago, NAPN combined with Safer Society Press, an excellent resource for books and treatment manuals related to working with people with sexual behavior problems. They also have training, webinars, links to information, and a podcast.

One of the first treatment manuals specifically written for adolescent male sex offenders, *Breaking the Cycle: Adolescent Sexual Treatment Manual*, was published in 1988. Several treatment manuals are available, some of which are aimed at specific populations. These include, but are not limited to, *Pathways*, *Roadmaps*, *Growing Beyond*, *Beacon*, and *Stages of Accomplishments*. It is important to remember that no treatment manual in and of itself is treatment on its own. I am aware of treatment programs that simply hand a workbook to the clients and have them fill it out and return it. That is not treatment. So far, I have only ever met one person who had been in legal trouble for their sexual behavior as a juvenile, was sent to treatment, and then reoffended as an adult. He was a graduate of a treatment program he had been ordered to as a juvenile. This program, which was in a secure facility, handed out workbooks to the youth and had them fill them out and return them. He reported to me that the boys in the program handed their answers down to each other over time and that the "work" they did in the book was just slightly modified copies of what previous clients had written in the past. There was no discussion of the treatment concepts or the clients' thoughts, feelings, or values. This young man got no benefit from his "treatment," and after he was released from the facility, he engaged in behavior nearly identical to what got him into trouble in the first place. Since he was an adult by that time, he entered the adult criminal justice system, which is how I met him. If he had received appropriate treatment the first time, he likely would have made different choices, and the person he victimized would not have had to endure that. It is imperative that treatment be well done to benefit the clients we are working with and prevent future risks to the community.

Working with court-ordered clients differs from working with clients who have voluntarily entered treatment. When working with a client who decided to come to therapy because it was their own desire to address something in their lives that was causing them distress, then that person is the client, and their best interests are the only focus. Forensic psychology can be thought of as clinical psychology in a legal setting. The involved nature of working with people who have been legally ordered to receive treatment moves us into forensic work, which has some important differences from typical therapy. When working with a person who was court-ordered to treatment because they engaged in harmful behavior, there is more than one "client" involved in the process. You have the court-ordered individual themselves. In addition, you generally have the referring agency, in other words, the court or county that sent the client to treatment, and you have community safety. It is very important that clients are aware of how that impacts treatment in the informed consent process and how it might be different if they were voluntarily seeking help for an area of concern. Court-ordered clients have the right to confidentiality just as clients who voluntarily enter therapy, but the circumstances differ. There are generally no confidentiality boundaries among the professionals who comprise the treatment team and the court. My court-ordered clients need to know that while I certainly will not talk about them to friends or family or random people on the street, probation officers, judges, and other treatment team members have access to their information. Even though clients are court-ordered, it is important for them to have all the informed consent information any other client would have and know that therapy is still a choice. While they probably will not like the consequences of choosing not to be in court-ordered therapy, it is still a choice they get to make. Occasionally I have had clients tell me that the nature of treatment was misrepresented to them by their lawyers, and if they had known what it was like, they would not have accepted their plea deal and would have taken jail or prison time. I always let them know that is an option. If they do not want to participate, they can simply have their lawyer or probation officer schedule a hearing and let the judge know their decision.

While most treatment programs use a treatment manual, it is important to realize that a well-done manualized treatment is not a cookie-cutter approach. Even if a treatment program uses the same treatment workbook for each client, the emphasis on specific assignments and chapters should be different for each individual. Depending on the client's individual treatment needs, material can be added or subtracted. Much of the work of treatment happens in discussing the information and the assignments. The assignments and information in whatever treatment manual is being used are a guide to covering the topics, and it is more important for treatment providers to keep in mind the individual needs of the clients they are working with, to focus solely and make sure every assignment in the book gets completed. Simply completing all the assignments in the treatment workbook is insufficient if the person has not made changes that reflect living in a healthy and low-risk way. The work of treatment can only happen within the context of a strong therapeutic relationship. No one wants to talk about their thoughts and feelings about things they have done that they feel shame about with someone they do not feel comfortable with. A strong therapeutic connection is necessary, though not sufficient on its own, for change to happen.

As mentioned earlier in this chapter, early research in sex offender treatment focused on incarcerated adult rapists and child molesters. That research, which did not generalize well to all adult offenders, was generalized to adolescent offenders and influenced early treatment programs. This resulted in many assumptions that were later proven false, and a lot of problematic treatment approaches developed. For example, the adults who participated in that early research generally reported that they had begun engaging in criminal sexual behavior when they were adolescents, so an assumption was made that all adult sex offenders begin abusing people while still young, which is not true, and that all adolescent offenders will go on to become adult sex offenders, which is also very much not true (Caldwell and Caldwell, 2022). More recent research has shown that the recidivism rate for juveniles who commit sex crimes is actually quite low (Laajasalo et al., 2020). Treating every child who engages in illegal sexual behavior as if they are destined to be an adult offender causes a great deal of harm. In addition, early research led to the false belief that all sex offenders have experienced sexual abuse themselves and that all offenders have multiple victims.

We now know that neither of these things is true. While many of the court-ordered clients I work with, both adults and youth, have experienced their own sexual abuse, many have not. In the same vein, while it is not unusual to learn that a client has had additional victims as they become more willing to be honest in treatment, it is also not unusual to find that they did not. Many early treatment programs focused on getting people to "confess" to having additional victims and to being survivors of abuse themselves, which is a problem when that is truly not the case for someone. I want my clients to be honest with me, and I do not want them to make stuff up because they think that is what I want to hear. In the past, some programs required clients to admit to additional victims to progress to the next level of the program, so youth would feel that they needed to make stuff up. A client in our program a while ago wanted to be "cool" in front of his peers and have to be the focus of attention and care, and he often made up stories about things he had been involved in. He once insisted he had witnessed a shooting while out with friends and that one of his friends had died in his arms. There had not been a shooting, and the friend was fine. My client just thought it was a good story to tell and that people would be nice to him if they thought he had just gone through a traumatic experience. Even without the pressure to confess to things to progress in treatment, I have worked with children who have told me they did things that they did not do because they thought that would ensure my attention or cause their parents to pay more attention to them. It is important that clients feel safe to be totally honest about their behavior and not feel like they have to make things up in order to be accepted.

Early treatment programs based on the false assumptions from the early adult research focused on shaming, confrontation, and strict adherence to rules with the idea of tearing people down in order to build them back up again. Current research shows that this approach does not work and is completely inappropriate. It does not work with adult offenders either, but it is especially problematic when working with youth. The more punitive in-your-face approach has led to putting even very young children on the sex offender registry, public notification, families that cannot reunite, young children being labeled as predatory, and children being unable to engage in typical childhood behaviors. Research has found that, just like in any other area of therapy, a strong therapeutic relationship is necessary for therapy to be effective. No one gets much out of treatment if their experience of it is someone yelling at them and treating them badly.

I do not know about you, but I do not have any desire or motivation to be open and vulnerable with someone who is treating me poorly and shaming me. There is no reason why we should think that would be helpful in any therapeutic context. It is not necessary or useful to treat people badly to try and help them make changes in their behavior. We cannot teach people, adults, or children to have good boundaries and treat others with respect and dignity if we are unwilling to model that in the way we interact with them. If I want you to learn how to treat people with dignity and respect, I need to show you how that behavior works when I am interacting with you and others. It is important for me to treat clients with dignity and respect no matter how they treat me. That doesn't mean that I don't have boundaries or would allow clients to be aggressive or overly rude; it just means I can enforce my boundaries while treating people respectfully. Often, clients and sometimes other professionals will talk about only treating people with respect when those people are also being respectful to them, stating things like "Respect is earned" or "I will treat you the way you treat me." I think this leads to a few problems. One is that if I am only going to be respectful to you if you are going to be respectful to me first, and you have the same thought, then neither of us will treat each other well, and we will both be too stubborn to break the pattern of interaction we have.

Another problem is that if a client is a person who has generally not seen respectful interaction modeled, it may be that even if they wanted to treat members of the treatment team with respect, they do not know how without someone showing them that behavior first. The third reason I think it can be problematic is that if I only treat others the way they treat me, I allow others to decide how I will behave. I would much rather decide how I would like to act rather than have other people's behavior control mine.

When I started working with adult offenders, the psychologist supervising me and the co-therapist in the groups I was in were male. I, by the way, am not. Some of the clients in those groups had never had a female therapist. One of the benefits of having both of us in a group was that the clients got to see how we interacted with each other and watched the male therapist treat a woman with dignity and respect. I will never forget one of the men in that group who said to me, during an individual session, with wonder and surprise, that he had just realized that women are a lot like men and have feelings like men do. It had honestly never occurred to this man that women also have feelings and that their feelings get hurt the way a man might. That is not an insight he would have been able to have if my colleague and I had spent his treatment time berating him.

Research has shown that most adolescents and adults who engage in sexually abusive behavior with young victims are not primarily sexually attracted to children. Of course, some individuals have a primary sexual attraction to children, but this is much rarer than people generally think. Often crimes against children are motivated more by access, anger, trauma, or power rather than just sexual attraction. That said, it is important to remember that arousal is a factor in sex crimes. After all, if it was just about power, without any sexual component, clients might have chosen to hit or scare the person in another way. I once worked with an adult client who had abused a girl in his neighborhood who used to come to his house, along with his grandchildren, after school. For a long time, my client insisted that the only reason he had abused this child was because he had caught her being abusive toward his grandchildren, and that was how he punished her. Once he was able to admit to himself that if the punishment was his only motivation, he would have grounded her, yelled at her, or banned her from his house or something similar, he was able to work through the shame he felt at the idea of having been aroused by a child. He was not a person whose primary sexual arousal was toward children, and his treatment mostly needed to focus on other things, but it was also important to note that sexual arousal was a component of the decisions he had made. Treatment programs that focus primarily on a client's deviant sexuality are not helpful if deviant sexuality is not an issue that is particularly problematic for the client. Sometimes an overfocus on deviance can leave people feeling like any sexual thought or feeling is bad, which just is not reasonable as most adolescents and adults have sexual thoughts and feelings very regularly. I have asked more than one teenager recently discharged from residential treatment what they should do if they see someone of the same age at school or in the community they think is cute or that they like. Often these youth will tell me that if that happens, they should look the other way, change their thoughts, and avoid the person. It seems odd to ask a teenager to never acknowledge that they might have feelings for another teenager and that if they do, it is bad, and they should avoid that person completely. A healthier approach is to discuss how to perhaps introduce oneself, ask for the other person's name, ask about the most recent homework assignment, etc. We want these clients to develop healthy relationships and healthy sex lives. To do that, they need to know how to talk to people they like and handle relationships and rejection appropriately. Telling them they just should not think about sex at all is not realistic or helpful. Treatment techniques that were designed to work with adults who struggle with deviant sexuality are not only not helpful for adolescents but also actively cause harm and are not an appropriate part of good quality treatment programs. Teaching youth how to recognize what is healthy and what is not healthy and how to handle unhealthy thoughts without shame is much more likely to get beneficial results for the client and the community.

Sex offender registration rules vary by state. While there are federal guidelines, like the Adam Walsh Act, not every state has adopted them, including the state I live in. The stated purpose of sex offender registration is community safety. However, it turns out that registries do not increase safety (Letourneau and Armstrong, 2008), and many professionals believe that they can increase risk (Harris et al., 2015). Different states, and even different counties, have different policies about registering youth. In some places, children, even some as young as ten years old, are being placed on the sex offender registry. In addition to public humiliation, this can make it nearly impossible for the families to find housing and may impact the child's ability to attend school and interact in the community. Increasing instability, isolation, and family stress is a great way to increase the risk for recidivism, but not at all useful in increasing community safety. In addition, harsh laws can lead to prosecutors being less likely to want to prosecute cases, so ironically, areas with harsher punishments for juveniles who commit sex crimes may find that fewer youth are held criminally responsible for their behavior (Letourneau et al., 2009).

While the field is still relatively new, we have made tremendous progress in the last little while, and through both clinical experience and juvenile-specific research, we have a much better idea of what works to help these young people get back on track. Just as children, in general, are not just little adults, current research has indicated that children with sexual behavior problems are not just small adult offenders. Treating juvenile offenders like adult offenders is inappropriate and unethical as their treatment needs differ. Children benefit from having "normal" social experiences while balancing community safety. That is one of the reasons why it is important to handle registration issues carefully. The recidivism rate for adolescent offenders is very low, and most do not become adult offenders. If we want these children to develop into functioning, healthy adults, we need to help them learn how to be functioning, healthy children with the skills to have healthy relationships and strong social support networks.

It is important to remember that treatment for juveniles with sexual behavior problems is a specialty. In Texas and some other states, providers are required to have a specialized license in order to be able to work with people who have gotten into legal trouble for their sexual behavior. In Texas, this is a secondary license. In other words, you already have to be a licensed mental health professional, like a psychologist, professional counselor, or clinical social worker. Then you can also become a licensed sex offender treatment provider (LSOTP). Some states have similar requirements, but even for other areas that do not, it is important to ensure that you get the appropriate training and supervision if you are working with this population. Research shows us that juveniles who commit sex crimes differ on many measures from those who commit other crimes.

Chapter 2

Youth in Treatment

When people hear the term "sex offender," even "juvenile sex offender," they get a certain picture in their minds. I remember someone I was talking to once who told me he would know if he was ever around a sex offender because he would just be able to tell if "that kind of a person" was near him. The truth was I was aware that he knew and hung out with someone who had that in their history, but of course, it would not have been appropriate for me to out the other person as an example of *not* being able to recognize that someone is a sex offender just by talking to them. I usually tell people that if they ever came to a group with me, they would find it really is just a roomful of people that look no different from any other type of meeting with a room full of people. That holds for both adults and youth. The youth I work with are just youth. They are youth who have behaved in ways that have caused a great deal of harm and who need help learning what was going on with them that contributed to them acting like that and how to make sure nothing like that ever happens again, but they are not fundamentally different than other children. Like all children, youth with sexual behavior problems need food, water, shelter, social interaction, positive attention, good role models, nurturing, appropriate structure, safety, and a good education. Community safety is very important, and so is the individual client's well-being and the family system in which they live. These things do not need to be in opposition, and community safety increases when the individual members and systems in the community are functioning well. The goals of community safety—no more victims, healing for the person who offended, and healing for the people the offender hurt—are goals that work well together and strengthen each other.

So who are these youth? There is no one answer to that question. Individuals who commit sex crimes come from all walks of life, economic backgrounds, types of family structures, religious backgrounds, and races and ethnicities. I usually work with youth who are in outpatient treatment and live in the community. While some of the youth who get in trouble for sexual behavior problems have also gotten in trouble for other law enforcement-related things, typically, most of the youth I work with have never been in trouble with the law before. The offense is often a big shock to their family and community. Some of my clients have been to or will need to go to residential treatment. Some need to be in a secure facility for a while, but overall, the youth I work with have been placed on probation and are living in the community while under a probation officer's supervision. Most of the information and stories in this book reflect that population. Often, youth in higher levels of care settings are there for a few reasons. Sometimes youth come from rural or isolated areas. No appropriate outpatient treatment providers are available in their community, so the judge routinely orders all youth who commit sex crimes in that area to residential or secure facilities. Sometimes clients show that they are not ready to be safe in the community, so while they may start as outpatient clients, it may become necessary to have a higher level of care for a while. Some clients are not a good fit for outpatient treatment. If, for example, their offense was very violent, a judge may decide it is too big of a risk to the community for that person to start their treatment in an outpatient setting. We have sometimes had to recommend inpatient settings for youth, not necessarily because of anything the adolescent was doing or not doing in outpatient treatment, but because the family was so chaotic or abusive, there were really no other safe alternatives. Some families do not have the capacity or sometimes the willingness to help support their youth through treatment and probation.

Many years ago, I worked with an adolescent whose parents decided to move out of state and leave him behind to complete his probation. When his parents left, they initially left him in the care of an older sibling; that person was a young adult but was in no way prepared to add a traumatized abandoned teenager with all the obligations probation and treatment bring to their already stressful life. The sibling was a lovely person and tried hard, but it was not a viable situation for either of them. Luckily our county had a halfway house facility that he could go to. He successfully completed outpatient treatment while living there and getting the support he needed from the staff. He kept in touch for many years after he graduated from treatment and is a husband, father, and functioning member of his community who, all these years later, still calls me to check in and let me know how things are going in his life. That halfway-house program later got eliminated, and a child in a similar situation in my county now would likely need to be placed in a residential treatment facility. Still, I am glad the safety net was there when he needed it, and I hope that option gets restored at some point. He sometimes struggled in treatment, but many of his struggles were not because of choices he was making but because of choices the adults in his life were making that he had no control over.

Youth in treatment are responsible for their own choices and doing what they need to do to be safe in the community, but we also need to keep in mind that they do not always have power over some of the choices made for them. A child who refuses to come to treatment or probation meetings or do any of the treatment assignments needs one kind of help and is often in a very different situation than a child whose parents cannot or will not bring them or who has so much chaos at home that there is not a time or place that they could do their treatment work.

Some of the youth we work with live in situations where they may not have any privacy to do treatment work, not always have enough food, or have unreliable utilities. Some of the youth we work with have adults struggling so much with their own trauma and issues that they do not have the capacity or sometimes the desire to be helpful to their children. Sometimes clients end up in higher levels of care facilities because the adults in their lives are unable or unwilling to support them. It is important to ensure that children are not punished for the choices the adults in their lives are making. In general, when it is possible, it is best to have children living at home in the community, but sometimes that is not a viable or safe option. For some youth, home is so stressful that being in a treatment facility feels better to them. On more than a few occasions, I have worked with youth who have told me they like being detained in the juvenile jail in our county. It is calmer there than at home. They know the rules and consequences and always have meals and a bed. It is heartbreaking to work with youth who find juvenile detention a nice break from dealing with what they have to deal with at home, but that is sometimes the case.

Nearly all the clients I see are on probation and court-ordered to sex offense-specific treatment. I also worked with youth who did not get prosecuted for their behavior, but their parents, foster parents, or residential or group home facility realized there was a problem and brought their youth for treatment voluntarily. It is difficult, however, to fully complete treatment when no outside authority is involved. In the county where I do most of my work, treatment costs for juveniles are almost always paid for by the county. Families who voluntarily engage in treatment have to cover the costs themselves or use their health insurance if possible, which can be prohibitive. They also do not always have access to the wraparound services, like mentors or family therapists, or food/clothing/transportation support that youth in the system often have.

The age varies from state to state, but in Texas, you can be as young as ten and be held legally responsible for your behavior. Sometimes I see youth with sexual behavior problems younger than ten, but that is usually because an adult in their lives has become concerned and wants them to get help before an existing problem worsens or causes more damage. Sometimes adults also overreact to behavior that is not developmentally unusual but makes them uncomfortable. Some of the younger youth are also court-ordered, not through the criminal justice system but the family court, as part of a judge's orders regarding a child in the foster care system. Most frequently, the youth I work with who have sexual behavior problems are boys, but I have worked with many girls. In addition to boys being more likely to engage in inappropriate sexual behavior than girls, they are more likely to be prosecuted, so I do not see many girls on probation. We usually have at least two or three court-ordered girls in our program at any given time. So while not as common as boys in treatment, it is also not unusual.

Like any other group of youth, children on probation have an array of intellectual functions. There are youth on probation for a sex offense of average or above-average intelligence who are not struggling with any intellectual, developmental, or academic disabilities. Some youth do have one or more issues that make a variety of things more difficult for them. Treatment plans should be individualized to the specific child and adjusted as the treatment team gets to know the child and their strengths and weaknesses better. It is not unusual for a youth's developmental maturity to be different from their chronological age, which can be a factor in social skills development. Those clients may need more or different interventions in that area. Some children have learning differences that make reading the treatment manual or writing their assignments more challenging. Some clients benefit from having the book read aloud for them or having the information presented in a way that best works for how they comprehend things. Some clients benefit from dictating their answers out loud instead of writing them or sometimes addressing treatment concepts through art or other media, allowing them to express themselves with less frustration. It is important that treatment and probation requirements be reasonable goals that the client has the capacity to achieve.

I am not a lawyer, and every state/county has different laws and rules, so what I see at work may be different from what you see or what is typical for the area near you. There are a few ways that youth get placed on probation and into treatment, and these often vary from state to state and sometimes even from county to county. Some youth are adjudicated, some have deferred adjudication, some start treatment while they are still pre-court, some are under a judicial confession, and some are in aftercare, which means they have already successfully graduated from a residential treatment program. The specifics of each type of legal situation are more impactful on the probation officer and the judge than on the treatment provider, with some exceptions. If a child is in treatment before the court process is complete, it is very important that the child and their family understand that treatment information can be used in court. Whenever I talk to families wanting treatment for their child, who has not yet gone to court or is still in the middle of the court process, I ask them to talk to their lawyer about it first. For treatment to work well, the client must be able and willing to be honest, so they need to know from their lawyers if it is okay to talk in therapy or if talking honestly would put them at legal risk. It might be better to wait until the court process resolves itself. The other category that impacts treatment is aftercare. Often youth who go to residential treatment are surprised and unhappy to graduate from that program only to find that the judge has ordered them to go to outpatient treatment as well. The reason for aftercare is that no matter how good the treatment quality is in a residential program, there is not much opportunity for the child to put their new skills into practice in the real world. Aftercare allows the client to work on treatment concepts that will be the most helpful in the real world and practice interacting with others while still having the support and monitoring of therapists, probation officers, and judges. An aftercare program may be shorter than a full treatment program, and a motivated youth could complete it in six months. That being said, the length of time a client takes in treatment is almost entirely based on the amount of time and effort they are willing to put in. Some youth who probably could have completed a typical aftercare program in six months drag it out for years. There are also youth in aftercare who do not appear to have benefited much from the residential program they were in and sometimes needed more comprehensive treatment than the standard aftercare program, so they can take longer.

31

Youth who engage in illegal sexual behavior come from all walks of life. Studies have shown that early childhood stressors and risk factors can contribute to the age of onset of the behavior (Adams et al., 2020). No one risk factor is absolutely predictive of who will commit a sex crime and who will not. There are several risk assessment tools on the market for juveniles, but all of them are designed to be used with youth who have already gotten in trouble for their sexual behavior. The tools are designed to predict the risk of recidivism, not first-time offenses. In addition, the tools currently on the market do not really do that great of a job in predicting behavior anyway. The literature on risk factors for recidivism is still relatively limited (Spice et al., 2013).

It is important for anyone using a risk assessment tool and for anyone reading a risk assessment report to remember that the diagnostic tools are flawed and should never be used on their own to make any pronouncements and that some of the tools were developed for research and treatment use and were not meant to end up being used in court in order to determine what happens to an individual. In addition, since children are growing and changing, no risk assessment on youth is valid for more than six months. I imagine as research continues, we will eventually have many more valuable tools on the market, but at the moment, what we do have needs to be used judiciously and cautiously, particularly regarding clients who are not in the populations the tools were normed on. It is also true that while risk assessment tools can be problematic and need to be used with caution, one should also be cautious of relying solely on clinical judgment, as research also shows us that professionals' individual attitudes toward offenders may lead to incorrect and possibly problematic decisions (Harper and Hicks, 2022).

Most youth who commit sex crimes do so with people who are important to them and are a regular presence in their lives, often younger siblings, stepsiblings, cousins, or close family friends. It cannot be very easy for families to figure out how to support all the children involved. Sometimes the judge keeps the youth together in the same home, and sometimes the adolescent who committed the offense needs to live elsewhere for a while. Often a grandparent, aunt, uncle, or other friend or relative will agree to allow the child on probation to live with them until they get to the point where the family can be reunited. It is helpful for treatment programs to include parent/guardian support and education. For example, parents or guardians of youth in treatment programs are often required to attend a monthly parent group (before the pandemic made groups problematic) and to complete chaperone training so that they can be involved in their child's treatment and have the tools they need to help maintain safety at home. The reoffense rate for juvenile sex offenders is very low, but very low does not mean zero.

The few times we have had a child in our program reoffend, it generally happens when the parents are unwilling to follow the guidelines we ask them to. That does not make the child any less responsible for their behavior, but it is an important reminder to the adults that they play a big role in their youth's success and the safety of everyone. Some adults are unable or sometimes unwilling to support their youth, and those youth have to navigate treatment essentially on their own. Treatment will usually take longer for those clients, and they may have more setbacks during the process. I have worked with many clients who were able to succeed in treatment and probation and go on to have safe lives despite having adults in their lives who were either unsupportive or sometimes even actively problematic. Some of the youth I work with have adults who are able and willing to be supportive, and those families can help make the treatment process as smooth as possible for everyone involved. By the time a child has gotten to a place in their life where they are willing to hurt another person in that way, often someone they love, there are usually lots of things going on. No matter how supportive the family is, youth in treatment will inevitably hit rough patches or have particular treatment concepts or assignments that they find very difficult to deal with. Expectations for youth and families in treatment should be clear and realistic. Some youths will take longer than others, and some youths have additional issues they need to work through, which may make completing treatment assignments less of a priority for a while. Effective treatment means addressing each client's individual needs and treating them as whole people with the dignity and respect every person deserves. Some programs have significant time constraints that can make addressing the child's needs more challenging. If it is logistically possible, it is beneficial when treatment professionals can work at the speed that is in the best interests of the individual child. Some youths go through it fairly quickly, and some do not, but I know that is a privilege that not all treatment providers have. That is another reason that aftercare can be very important for youth who have had residential treatment. They have the chance to practice living safely in the real world and the space to process and deal with issues that might not have been addressed in the residential program, many of which have more time constraints than I usually have in outpatient treatment.

Chapter 3

Components of a Good Treatment

W hat components would help ensure that a treatment program is of high quality and that the clients who are part of it get the best, most useful therapy they can? The program's content is important—a sexual behavior treatment program that only consisted of cooking classes would not be particularly useful—but the way the program approaches treatment is more important than the specific content they focus on. A program can have the best content available, but the content would not do any good if the providers are shaming, dismissive, and condescending toward the clients. No program will work well without a good therapeutic approach and providers who can foster healthy, appropriate therapeutic relationships with the clients.

From everything I knew about a chemistry teacher I had in high school, it appeared he had lots of knowledge about chemistry to share. Unfortunately, he was rude, condescending, and dismissive, especially toward female students. I learned very little in class that year about chemistry. What I did learn, however, was to keep my head down and never ask him questions when I was confused about something. The content of his class was drowned out by his approach to teaching. Luckily a good knowledge of high school chemistry was not necessary to successfully navigate high school. While I found being in his class stressful and annoying, my inability to be successful in his class did not impact my or anyone else's safety or freedom to live in the community. It did, however, contribute to me not taking any college chemistry classes, but since I was a psychology major, that also had no significant long-term impact on me.

The impact of not being successful in a sex offense-specific treatment program is much more profound. Those who are unsuccessful in treatment may get ordered to residential or secure facilities. They may be required to be on the sex offender registry, reoffend sexually or nonsexually, and not figure out how to have healthy relationships and good boundaries. Those are much more serious consequences than simply not liking or knowing much about chemistry. It is vitally important that clients be given the tools and the space they need to succeed in treatment to be successful in the community.

While I will be using this section to talk about the qualities that are important in treatment providers, court-ordered clients have a team of professionals involved in their treatment, and everyone involved must treat the clients and each other with dignity and respect and model the characteristics that increase client success. As therapists and other professionals, you have a lot of power, and you must recognize that and be able to demonstrate to the client that you are trustworthy and that you will not abuse your power. Court-ordered clients often have little to no choice about who their treatment provider or probation officer is. They are also coming in for treatment, having just gone through the court process, which is stressful and overwhelming. Shortly before their therapy intake appointment, they met with their probation officer, got a long list of rules they needed to follow, and were told about all the consequences if they did not do what they were supposed to do. The family has just learned that they will need permission from probation to do many things they would like to do and have sometimes been told that already planned trips and events may not be possible. Now they get to meet with a therapist who wants to ask them lots of questions about the most shameful and overwhelming time in their lives and also lets them know they have even more rules to follow and that they need to be very honest, even though they are being asked to talk to a complete stranger about deeply personal stuff. I have met many clients who were told by their lawyers that treatment was not a big deal, something that would be brief, and would not take a lot of effort on their part. When those clients discover the extent of what treatment entails, they are often pretty overwhelmed and unhappy and report feeling lied to by the people involved in their legal case.

Clients are aware that as their therapist, you will talk to their probation officer, and if they mess this treatment stuff up, they might have to go back in front of the judge and possibly have major consequences. This dynamic is often compounded further if the client is a member of a marginalized population historically treated poorly by the justice and medical/mental health systems, especially if the professionals involved are not from the same or even another marginalized population. While treatment works best if the client is honest, it is essential that all professionals involved be realistic with allowing clients and families time to settle into being on probation and treatment and get to know the professionals who are now in their lives. Many of my clients come to treatment feeling defensive and with a lot of secretiveness and worry. The vast majority of them calm down after a bit and participate actively. It is unrealistic to expect them to trust and feel comfortable with their treatment providers from day one. Many families also value family loyalty, and children are sometimes told not to discuss certain things in therapy. I have worked with many clients who have gotten into trouble at home because they have discussed something in treatment that their parents did not want other people to know.

Of course, when working with children, you are also working with their families. All the stress and worry that the child is feeling is also being felt by the adults, who are often worried that the professionals involved will think they are bad parents and possibly take their children away. In many cases, the parents of the child who offended are also the parents of the victim, and they are struggling to support both or all of their children. In some cases, this means managing to have their children live in two separate households. Families may be balancing treatment appointments, probation appointments, court hearings, therapy appointments for their other children, and sometimes therapy appointments for themselves, along with all the usual tasks of day-to-day living. This is an overwhelming situation for adults who have jobs that do not allow for flexibility or do not have reliable transportation. Many of the parents have their own trauma. It is not unusual for them to have experienced sexual abuse themselves, so sometimes the content of treatment-related conversations can be difficult for them to cope with.

Compassion and realistic expectations are important. The foundation of treatment is a safe relationship. When I started working as an intern, I worked primarily with adult offenders. A gentleman in one of the groups would not speak directly to me about any of his therapy assignments or really about anything else most of the time. If my supervisor (and co-therapist) stepped out of the room, he would stop participating in the group and wait for him to come back into the room. He told me once that it was not that he did not like me. He just trusted my supervisor's level of education more than he trusted mine. This went on for a long while. One day we had to abruptly cancel the group because of bad weather. He was already at the office and needed to head back home. He was a person who was not comfortable with change or deviations in his expected routine, so before he left, I reminded him to drive carefully and take his time to be safe on the way home, as he would likely be tense because of the unexpected change. We talked briefly about perhaps taking a breath and relaxing before heading out, especially since he was driving while the weather was bad. The following week he started treating me the same way he treated the therapists he had been working with longer, and he told me that when I told him to drive carefully, it demonstrated to him that I cared about him and that he could trust me. In the end, it was not really that my degree was not as prestigious as he would have liked. He just needed to feel safe and comfortable in the therapeutic relationship. I could have had the best therapeutic techniques and content in the world, but that did not matter half as much as my telling him to drive carefully in bad weather and him realizing that I knew him well enough to know the change in his routine would especially stress him and that I cared about his well-being. Like all other humans, clients want to feel comfortable with the people they interact with, and until they do, it will be difficult for them to move forward in treatment.

What creates a relationship that feels safe? In some ways, to answer that question, we just need to think about what goes into us feeling comfortable with the people we interact with. Of course, the therapeutic relationship differs from a relationship with a friend, co-worker, or family member. Still, some of the underlying characteristics that make us feel safe and comfortable with others are the same things that help clients feel safe in the therapeutic relationship. In the therapeutic relationship and relationships with probation officers and other professionals, it is also important to remember that a power differential exists and that the onus of creating safety in the relationship is on the treatment provider or other professional, not the client.

Some important factors include focused attention, understanding of the person's unique context, nonjudgmental approaches, empathy, and trustworthiness. Therapists who are respectful, flexible, warm, affirming, understanding, interested, and honest help contribute to positive therapeutic alliances necessary for good client outcomes.

Working with clients who have committed a sex crime is not all that different from working with other clients who come to therapy for other reasons. All clients want to feel safe, heard, respected, and understood. Most therapists are aware of the importance of active listening, paying attention to nonverbal cues, and checking in to make sure that the person is being understood and is understanding you. The good communication and listening skills that are the foundation of any therapeutic relationship are also the foundation of therapeutic relationships with court-ordered clients. While there are definitely differences between working with a court-ordered person and a client who has sought out therapy independently, the fundamental skills are the same. They should not be forgotten or abandoned simply because the client is legally required to be there, and treatment is forensic in nature.

As was mentioned earlier, court-ordered clients come from all walks of life. That is true of adult offenders and youth with sexual behavior problems. It is important to learn about who that person is and what they as an individual need and want and to meet them where they are. I am surprised at the number of times I have met with young children in treatment programs designed for adults that required them to behave like an adult. An eleven-year-old who committed a sex crime is still only eleven years old and should not be expected to succeed in a treatment program originally designed for adults. That program would not only not be helpful, but it would likely also cause harm to the client. Some of the youth who come to treatment are developmentally delayed or have other challenges and should also be treated accordingly. If you have a treatment program that is very writing or reading-heavy and you do not make accommodations for clients with learning differences or other developmental or educational issues, then you are setting up your clients for failure, and that is not okay. It is imperative to approach the client as a whole person who needs help changing their behavior, not just as the behavior that happens to be attached to a person. It is also important not to criminalize normal developmental behavior. I have met youth who have come out of treatment programs with the idea that any time they have any sexual thoughts about anyone, they must immediately stop those thoughts. If they do not, it is problematic and an indication of deviance or a potential crime. Of course, in the real world, teenagers are going to have sexual thoughts, they are going to be attracted to other youth at school, and they are going to want to date. Teaching youth that normal teenage thoughts, feelings, and behaviors are problematic is confusing for them and sets them up to lie in therapy and perhaps have significant social interaction problems as they get older. Clients must learn how to recognize which sexual feelings are typical and which are problematic and how to handle their sexual feelings safely and responsibly. They cannot do that if they do not feel comfortable and safe enough to acknowledge and talk about their thoughts and feelings.

Flexibility is an important component of meeting people where they are. When I first started working as an intern, a man in one of our adult groups had undergone an organ transplant. He was on a lot of medication to help keep his body from rejecting the organ, which made him significantly immunocompromised. He was often not able to attend a group.

When I saw him for individual sessions, I kept him updated about my and my immediate family's health so that he would know if someone close to me was ill and could make informed decisions about protecting his own health. We would sometimes need to reschedule if any illness might impact him. I found out later that before being in our treatment program, he had been discharged from his original treatment program and identified as someone who refused to participate in treatment. The treatment providers in his original program required all their clients to attend both group and individual sessions and did not excuse most absences. While it is ideal for clients to regularly attend group and individual sessions, that would have put this man's life at risk and was not a reasonable expectation for him to follow. Luckily his probation officer and the judge gave him a chance to try with a different treatment provider rather than incarcerating him, which besides being not useful from a treatment perspective, would have been detrimental to his health. He was able to be successful in treatment. I ran into him in public many years later, and he let me know that he and his longtime partner were married and had two little boys whom I got to meet. He completed his treatment almost two decades ago and has been living safely and successfully in the community. While it is necessary to require court-ordered clients to follow treatment rules and expectations, both so they can get what they need out of treatment and to ensure community safety, it is also important to keep in mind these are people with real-world issues in their lives that do not just go away because it is not convenient for the treatment providers. Many of the youth I work with are involved in extracurricular activities at school. Sometimes practices, games, performances, field trips, etc., are scheduled simultaneously as therapy sessions. It is important that as much as is safely possible, youth have the chance to participate in typical teenage activities. It is important to find a good balance between making sure the clients get what they need from treatment and also getting what they need for the rest of their lives as well. For some youth, that does mean being able to miss or be late for sessions in order to go to sports practices during the sports season. For some youth, it is more important that they attend all their sessions and worry about sports or whatever activity they are interested in at a different time. Flexibility and treating the child as a whole person are key in making decisions about those kinds of activities.

Nearly all clients who go to therapy, for whatever reason, are at least a little worried about being judged. Individuals court-ordered into therapy because of their behavior are usually very worried about being judged. This can sometimes lead to initial hostility and defensiveness, which can be off-putting to others. Shame is an overwhelming debilitating feeling and can make it very difficult for someone to learn, heal, and grow. I remember an intake appointment I had several years ago with a court-ordered adult client. When the session was over, I told him I would see him at his next appointment, and I was glad to have met him. He turned to me and said, "No, you're not." He told me that since he was a sex offender, no one was glad to meet him, and no one would ever want to talk to him or have anything to do with him again. His shame made it difficult for him to believe anyone would want to have anything to do with him and made it hard for him to believe what I said, even if it was just a simple "Nice to meet you." That shame made it hard for him to imagine a future for himself. He worked through that and ended up being very successful in treatment and safe in the community. His outcome might have been very different if he had been in a judgmental or shame-based treatment program.

Another important component of therapy is the client's motivation. When I was in school, professors often talked about the need for a client to be motivated, some of them saying or at least implying that therapy with clients compelled to be there would not be useful as those clients were not motivated to change. I have found that that is not necessarily the case. Of course, eventually, clients must want to get some benefit from treatment, but I have worked with many individuals who initially only wanted to show up often enough that the judge would not get mad and they could get through probation and on with their lives. In the beginning, many clients are motivated by their desire to stay out of jail and not get into further trouble rather than feeling a need or desire to change. The vast majority of these individuals eventually buy in and become invested in the process, especially once they start noticing some positive impacts in their lives. In some ways, working with court-ordered clients is not that different from working with other youth whose parents require them to come to therapy though they do not want to. They have the same level of motivation in the beginning, just bigger consequences if they do not eventually buy in. Of course, with enough threats, power, and leverage, almost anyone can be compelled to do almost anything, but that is not really useful from a treatment perspective. It is important to help clients develop internal motivation. They will not be on probation forever, and if their only motivation for making safe choices is the leverage and power of the adults around them, there is no reason for them to continue making safe choices when the threat of probation or court consequences is removed. So how does one help a cranky hostile youth, a depressed, unmotivated youth, or a terrified, timid youth find the motivation to truly acknowledge and take responsibility for their behavior and do what it takes to heal and grow? Many factors can help; patience, the ability to avoid power-struggling, giving youth and families as much choice as possible, having a sense of humor, and using the principles of motivational interviewing. Many books are written on motivational interviewing, and many different types of training are available. I am not planning on going in-depth about it here, but it is an approach that emphasizes meeting the client where they are at and helping them find their own motivation and goals.

For example, many years ago, I had a young adult client (not court-ordered) who drank a lot and often drove when drunk. He was not particularly interested in stopping that behavior and told me he thought it would be strange not to go out and get drunk most days, and he did not understand people who did not drink to get drunk. The idea that someone would go out and only have one drink, or perhaps not drink, baffled him. He was also convinced that being drunk did not impact his driving ability. My disagreement with that had no impact on his behavior. However, he wanted to keep his job and could see the connection between drinking on the nights before he worked and getting into trouble at work for being late, cranky with customers, or absent altogether. The important factor to him was not to drink less but to retain his job. With that motivation, he concluded that it would work better for him if he did not go out drinking on nights when he had work the next day. He also concluded that misplacing his car or getting arrested again for driving while intoxicated also impacted his ability to be at work. It would be better to drink at home or make sure he had a ride planned. Again, his motivation had nothing to do with the morality or legality of driving drunk. His motivation to stop that behavior came from wanting to stay employed. The results were the same, though. When he had more days that he did not drink, he also started to notice that he felt better and had more money, time, and energy for other things he wanted to do. Eventually, he started talking about cutting back on his drinking more significantly. When he and I started talking about the topic, I wasted some time and energy trying to convince him that the amount he was drinking was bad for his health and that driving drunk was dangerous for him and everyone around him. He was used to being lectured by other people and easily dismissed my thoughts on the subject. When we started looking at his own thoughts, he found the internal motivation to make some changes in his behavior. That happens with court-ordered clients too. After being in treatment for a while, a client will often come to a session and say with surprise that they used something they learned in treatment in a real-world interaction with someone in their lives. The situation went better than similar situations had in the past. Once individuals start noticing that they get some benefits, they become more invested in the process.

Treatment programs should have multiple ways to measure the progress that the clients are making. Many programs are divided into phases of treatment, and of course, one way of measuring progress is if clients move through each phase and on to the next one at a reasonable rate of speed. Usually, moving from one phase to the next involves completing the treatment assignments, and of course, while important, treatment assignments are not the only measure of progress. A client's level of honesty is also one of the markers that can be measured for progress. Clients are often not completely honest, especially when they first start treatment. A growing willingness to be honest and to take responsibility for their choices is a positive sign. Often clients get overwhelmed when dealing with difficult issues, topics, or concepts that they find overwhelming. Sometimes youth will get very angry whenever a particular topic arises, or sometimes very avoidant of particular topics or assignments. Many of the individuals in treatment do not initially have the skills needed to manage conversations about topics they find difficult. Increased willingness to deal with difficult topics and an increased ability to manage and tolerate frustration and distress is another good indication of treatment progress.

I used to facilitate a treatment group for girls with sexual behavior problems living at a residential treatment facility. Often during group, at least one of the girls would say, "Miss, you are bringing up my issues," or comment that they had uncomfortable feelings because of the topic of conversation. We had many discussions in that group about managing big feelings and the possibility of sitting with feelings and using healthy coping skills as an option instead of throwing their books down and running out of the room. One of the ways we measured progress with those girls was their growing ability to stay in the room during group and to be able to talk about and manage their feelings, especially when that increased distress tolerance was also evident in other areas of their lives. Of course, attendance or lack thereof can indicate how a client is doing in treatment. As discussed earlier, it is important to look at the whole picture. If a child has poor attendance, the lack of attendance may say more about the parents' choices than the child's—a twelve-year-old with no access to transportation depends upon their parent or guardian to bring them.

Similarly, if the parents do not have access to reliable transportation, lack of attendance may be more of a situational/logistical problem than an indicator of commitment to treatment from either the parent or the child. Of course, a level of participation in treatment is essential. Some youth are naturally more comfortable talking than others, but eventually, it is good if all of them are willing to share feedback and comments in group.

I said earlier that while most treatment programs use workbooks, the workbook on its own is not treatment. If a client completes all the assignments in the book but hangs out unsupervised with young children or is looking at pornography regularly, they have not made much progress despite working on the book. It is not fair to judge a client on family participation, but the way a family handles supervision, rules, and participation can be an indication of how much support the youth has at home and how easy or difficult it will be for them to stay safe when they return home from residential treatment or when their term of probation is over, and they are in the community without the supervision and support of probation officers and treatment providers. Parents can also give another perspective on how the child behaves at home and in the community. Sometimes the first indication of a problem or that the youth is improving can be feedback from parents who talk about how things are going at home.

Multiple sources of information are always better than just one. Probation officers see the youth under different circumstances than treatment providers and can provide useful information about how the child is doing. Often probation officers will notice something in the home that can help give a much more accurate picture of what is going on with an adolescent. For example, a young man in treatment struggled a lot with pornography, and he would watch it whenever he could on any device that he could. The behavior was such a problem that he had a rule that he could only use a computer if his parent was sitting right there looking at the screen. The client reported that was what was happening, and the parent also reported that was what was happening, and for a while, it was. When visiting the youth at home, the probation officer noticed that the computer's monitor was turned slightly and where the mom was sitting did not provide that clear of a view. That info helped lead us to being able to talk to him about what was going on, and he admitted that he had slowly manipulated the setup so that his parent had not noticed the change, but that allowed him to look at whatever he wanted without being observed. The parent was not lying to us, and they really thought they were monitoring their child. This young man was just very good at manipulation. Multiple sources of information help keep things from slipping through the cracks.

The length of time in treatment will also vary from program to program and from client to client. Sometimes time in treatment is determined by the particular type of program the client is in. Some programs last a specific length of time, while others are more flexible. Different treatment programs have different goals, and sometimes the specific goals for treatment ordered by the court can vary from client to client, impacting how long treatment will take. Other factors that can impact the time a client is in treatment include family secrecy. Sometimes parents or other family members will instruct a child not to tell their therapist about things going on at home, making it difficult for the child to progress. The level of family chaos also has a big influence. Some of the youth we work with do not know from day to day where they are going, which adults they will be with, and what is expected of them. It is hard for youth living in chaos to focus on anything else, school and treatment included. The level of early childhood trauma and current trauma and stressors also impact the amount of time youth need in treatment. Many youths have high levels of shame, making progress in treatment difficult for them. Of course, neurological and learning differences also impact how long an individual child will need to meet their treatment goals.

What therapeutic approaches are the most common and useful when working with people with sexual behavior problems? As mentioned above, interpersonal connection and therapeutic relationships are among the most important factors. Assuming that is in place, many programs use a combination of therapeutic approaches and theories. The most common are cognitive behavioral therapy (CBT), relapse prevention, self-regulation theory, attachment theory, trauma-informed approaches, risk-need-responsivity, good lives model, dialectical behavior therapy (DBT), mindfulness, and restorative justice. Some programs emphasize one or more of these things more

49

than others, but most programs have at least some components of most of the above.

Many programs emphasize some form or forms of mindfulness and self-monitoring. Clients benefit from learning to both identify their emotions and be able to manage and cope with them. It is important that individuals learn how to be aware of their impulses, identify if those impulses are safe or not, and have coping skills to help manage inappropriate or unsafe ones. Many treatment programs also emphasize recognizing patterns or cycles of behavior and identifying how current behavior is impacted by things that happened in the past. As clients learn to be aware of their behavior patterns, they can also learn to recognize and step out of patterns and cycles that lead to problematic behavior. Overall, a big component of most treatment programs is psychoeducation, in other words teaching youth about what is healthy and what is not, how to identify and create healthy relationships in their lives, and how their own and their families' thoughts, feelings, and values impact them. However, knowledge alone is not enough. I can know that I would like to build a table, and I can know that I need wood and nails and tools and such, but that does not mean I will be able to produce a table since I have no furniture-making skills. I can guarantee that my having the materials and the desire would still not lead to a nice-looking table. It is important that treatment programs also emphasize skill-building and that clients learn and practice taking responsibility, communicating well, setting their own and respecting others' boundaries, managing their own feelings, and being aware of other people's feelings as well. The relative importance of any given skill or set of skills will depend on the individual client and his or her needs. Treatment should be individualized to the client. Individual clients respond well to individualized approaches, even when using treatment manuals.

Clients benefit when treatment providers can both maintain structure and provide flexibility.

Chapter 4

Treatment Team

Ideally, working with court-ordered clients with sexual behavior problems involves a team approach. The specific members of the team will vary depending on the specific circumstances, the type of treatment facility, the particular jurisdiction, and the needs of the individual client. Treatment teams generally include the youth and their adults, the treatment provider(s), the probation officer(s), and often a polygrapher. In addition, teams may include the judge and other court officials, case managers, other therapists involved with the client and their family, the victim's therapist, mentors, residential treatment staff, lawyers, and other professionals involved in the case. A team approach is good, but it only works well if everyone involved knows and sticks to what their roles are. The probation officer's role includes enforcing conditions of probation, monitoring and possibly restricting the client's activities, supervising, responding to violations, and rewarding progress. The role of the polygrapher is to monitor honesty in treatment, which helps with denial and helps ensure an accurate sexual history, leads to more useful and individualized treatment plans, and helps assess compliance with probation conditions. The district attorney is the legal representation of the community and the individual victims, and the judge makes decisions about placement and consequences. Treatment providers range from the person (or people) who provide the sex offense-specific treatment to other providers who may offer family therapy, mentors, case management services, etc.

The treatment provider should not try to do things that are the probation officer's job, and the probation officer should not try to be the treatment provider. If everyone sticks to their roles, things go much more smoothly. I have often worked with clients who are also working with other therapists and often for a specific issue they wish to address separately. Generally, this works very well. Over the years, I have had clients working with other therapists who insist on working on some of the sex offense-specific issues that the client is coming to treatment for, which has never gone well, as that is not their role with the client. I remember a child whose other therapist had him bring his sexual behavior problem treatment book to her sessions, and they would work on it together. The problem was that this therapist was unfamiliar with sex offense-specific therapy and often gave this client feedback and advice contradictory to what we were doing in treatment. He would sometimes bring incorrectly done work in but insist it was correct as it was what his other therapist told him to do. Her role officially was as a family therapist to work on the relationship he and the uncle who was raising him had. Unfortunately, her unwillingness to stay within her role and area of expertise did harm to our client and his family. It also likely contributed to her missing signs of significant problems. As it turned out, this child needed to be removed from that uncle because he was abusing him and denying him food.

In another case, I was working with a youth in a residential treatment facility due to a Child Protective Services situation, not her own behavior. The plan was to transition her home, and the family had a therapist who was supposed to be helping the family through that process. Rather than focus on that, the family therapist mostly met individually with my client and spent a great deal of time shaming her and requiring her to talk about things with her siblings that neither she nor her siblings were ready to discuss. That therapist also ended up doing a great deal of harm. It is very important that everyone involved in a case be clear about their roles and stick to them throughout the process. It is also important that treatment team members communicate with each other. In both the cases I mentioned earlier, with other therapists who complicated a situation needlessly, neither of those people was willing to discuss the situation with the rest of the treatment team.

What makes a good treatment provider? There has been a lot of research looking at what makes therapy successful. Much of that information is referenced in other sections of this book. Therapists who work with court-ordered clients should have the same therapeutic qualities important to all therapists. What makes a good probation officer? As far as I know, there is not nearly as much research about what qualities are important in a probation officer as there is about what qualities are important in a therapist. Many of the same principles apply, however. Especially when working in juvenile probation, officers need to understand child and adolescent development. It is important not to set youth up to fail by having expectations that are not reasonable and do not take typical teenage development into account. When working with children with special needs or challenges, it is useful for probation officers to know the reasonable expectations for that individual child. Of course, being trauma-informed is important for everyone who works with this population. For a lot of the public, working with people who have committed a sex crime is off-putting, and it is important that anyone who works with this population be able to keep in mind the whole human being involved, not just the crime. Many years ago, one of the juvenile probation officers I worked with approached me after a staffing meeting. He told me that he found reading the offense descriptions in the youths' files very disturbing and worried that his reaction to the offenses impacted how he treated the youth. He was a great probation officer, and the youth did not feel shamed or attacked by him, but the effort it took to deal with what he read in the file negatively impacted him and his well-being. He moved to a different area in probation and worked with youth with other types of crimes. I admire his self-awareness, willingness to ask for help, and willingness to make a change to protect his mental health and the well-being of the youth he worked with. Working with people who commit sex crimes is not for everyone, and it is important to realize if it is not for you to move on to something else.

Communication between probation officers and treatment providers is important. In the county I typically work with, we generally have a staffing meeting once per month attended by the probation officers and the providers. We discuss all the clients in the program. In addition, it is not unusual for me to exchange fairly frequent emails, phone calls, or texts with the probation officers of the youth I am working with. For example, a fairly new client in our program was not being totally honest with me about an event that he went to. His probation officer was at that event and had contacted me to let me know that he was there and what he was doing while he was there. Our communication helped the family and the client as there was not as much opportunity for them to lie about the situation. Once they were honest, they could more easily talk about what they had been thinking and why they made the choices they made.

One thing that often surprises other professionals is that the probation officers we work with typically attend groups at least once per month. That practice halted because groups stopped due to the pandemic; however, once we return to having groups, we will resume having probation officers sometimes join us. One year at a conference, the probation officers from our county presented about their sex offense-specific unit and how they work. When they talked about attending the group, there was a strong reaction from the people in the audience. Many treatment providers in the room felt strongly that having probation officers come to the group would disrupt the group dynamic, make it difficult for the clients to feel comfortable, and invade the therapeutic relationship. I can understand their reaction; however, we have found that, in actuality, the opposite has been true. In all the years that I have been doing groups that are visited by probation officers, I have only seen it be problematic one time in an adult group, and that was specific to that particular officer, and the way she viewed and approached things and the style of treatment and probation she worked in.

Typically youth are excited to see that their probation officer is in the group. More often, I get complaints from them if they feel like their specific probation officer is not visiting the group often enough. The youth enjoy showing off how they are doing and their progress. They benefit from the probation officers' understanding of how a group works and what we typically do. Since probation officers see the youth in a wider range of settings than treatment providers typically do, they can also let us know if an adolescent acts very differently at home than they do in the office, and that can help us know if things are going on that may be causing the child problems. Several years ago, the probation officers in our county also started offering study group time at the probation office where youth could come to work on their book assignments. Some of our youth do not have privacy or a calm space at home to get anything done, and this gives them space and the supervision of adults who care about their well-being. Since the probation officers supervising the study time had been in groups and seen most of the assignments presented, they could also answer most of the questions from clients who were confused about something. Those study times stopped because of the pandemic, but they were useful for the youth when possible. Though probation officers are sitting in group, the idea that the treatment team works best when we all maintain our own roles still applies. Probation officers are not there as extra therapists but are there in their role as probation officers. Most of the time, the probation officers I have worked with do not participate too much, except perhaps to add any announcements they might have at the beginning when we make general announcements. Some individuals do participate more than others. A probation officer used to come monthly to an adult group I ran in a more rural county in Texas. He often made comments or asked questions in the group, sometimes even sharing about things that had happened in his life.

Interestingly, the clients enjoyed having him and were disappointed when his schedule changed, and he could not join us anymore. He was only the officer for a few of the clients, but even the ones who had other officers enjoyed getting to know him and showing off their progress and knowledge when he came to the group. They were happy to have an officer who understood what treatment was like, and his participation in some of the group discussions humanized him and made them feel more connected to him. As long as all interactions with the probation officer come from a place of humanity and respect, it appears to benefit everyone involved. As I mentioned, the one problematic officer in the group was very shaming in her interactions with the clients and had difficulty sticking to her role. She only attended one group, and since it was a problematic experience for the clients, she was not invited back. The group was able to process that experience, and it did not harm the therapeutic relationships that had already been established.

It is crucial for all members of the treatment team to be sure they are aware of their own stress levels and triggers. We spend much of our professional time delving into the world of sexual violence and trauma. If professionals are not careful, they can find themselves burnt out, overly stressed, and traumatized. Most of our work is confidential, so we cannot go home and talk to our friends and family about work, and often what we deal with at work would disturb other people anyway. It is important to find outlets and ensure that you are monitoring your own stress levels. You will not be helpful to the clients if you do not have any energy left to give.

Often abuse happens within a family, and sometimes those families want to work toward reunification. The process of clarification and reunification can be complicated and has its own chapter later in the book. When reunification is the goal, it is important that the person (or people) who were victimized also have a therapist willing to be involved in the reunification process. Not all therapists or agencies are comfortable with the idea of reunification. I have known many abused children who wanted to reunify but had to change therapists as their original therapist was not comfortable participating in that process, or they worked for an agency whose policies prohibited it. If the victimized person has a good relationship with their therapist and has to change to someone else to reunify, that can be a big loss for them. Whenever possible, if clarification or reunification is likely to be a goal, it is helpful to choose a therapist who is open to that possibility.

Chapter 5

Polygraph Exams

Few things in the world of sex offense-specific treatment generate more controversy among treatment providers than discussions about the use of polygraph exams. In some places, they are considered a standard part of most treatment programs. They are viewed as problematic assessments that should never be used in other places. As with many things, I believe that the issue has more nuance than is usually discussed and that hard lines on either side of the debate can miss aspects of the issue.

In Texas, where I am located, polygraph use is an expected part of treatment programs. The ethics code of our licensing board (the Council on Sex Offender Treatment or CSOT) lists polygraph as one of the components treatment programs are supposed to contain. In 2017 the Association for the Treatment of Sexual Abusers (ATSA) put out practice guidelines for treating juveniles that recommended against using polygraph exams. In response, many programs in various parts of the country limited or stopped using polygraph exams completely.

There are a few reasons that polygraph exams are controversial. Few research studies look at polygraph use with juveniles, so there is not much evidence-based data to turn to for answers. Many individuals also feel that using a polygraph is coercive, as the clients are required to take them. I find that objection a little odd, given that the entirety of court-ordered treatment is coercive. Our clients usually participate in treatment because they are ordered to by a judge, and the consequences for not participating, usually incarceration, are something they want to avoid. There are many requirements, like curfews, community service, probation meetings, travel restrictions, etc., that clients likely only comply with to avoid the consequences that would occur if they chose to violate their court-ordered rules and expectations. Other assessments are often used to make decisions about an individual's treatment plan. These include but are not limited to psychosexual, neuropsychological, risk, and psychiatric assessments. The other assessment tools are often not as controversial as the polygraph exam, though many do not have very convincing bodies of research to reference.

Perhaps one of the reasons why polygraph exams have a controversial reputation is, in part, because people do not have a good understanding of what they are, the different types of polygraph exams, the different uses for polygraph exams, how to tell if someone has conducted a good quality exam, and how to use them appropriately. Some people do not treat polygraph exams as a treatment assessment tool but use them as a law enforcement tool. That is not how polygraphs should be used in therapy programs for young people with sexual behavior issues. Like any other assessment tool used in mental health, the polygraph is not a stand-alone tool, and decisions should not be made based solely on one assessment. Like many other assessments used in therapy, a polygraph can be a valuable and important component of looking at the whole picture of an individual client and their treatment progress.

There are four types of polygraph exams to work with people with sexual behavior problems. These four types are *the instant offense*, *sexual history*, *maintenance*, and *monitoring*. Each type serves a different purpose and should not be combined when doing a polygraph exam. A qualified polygraph examiner should administer polygraph exams, and when working with people with sexual behavior problems, the examiner should have specialized training in that field.

In Texas, a polygrapher who wants to work with people in legal trouble for a sex crime must be on the Joint Committee of Offender Testing (JPCOT) roster to do that type of work. The roster, which is kept and updated by the polygraph association of this state, has a list of those examiners that have the proper training and attend twenty hours of continuing education every two years. Not every client is a good candidate for a polygraph exam, and an appropriately trained and licensed polygrapher will be able to determine if a polygraph will be a useful assessment tool for the specific individual. Every state and every licensing board has some differences. The ethical code for the *Council of Sex Offender Treatment in Texas* states, "The polygraph examiner is the authority in determining if a polygraph examination is appropriate for a juvenile" (chapter 810.67 8E).

It is important to remember that while polygraphs are often called "lie detector" tests, they do not measure truth and lies. They measure deception. So if a client says something that is factually untrue but is also something they truly believe, they will pass the exam. If a client is deceptive, they will not pass the exam. It is also important to remember that the client may indicate deception on a question, not necessarily because of what the question specifically asks but because they are deceptive about something related to it. For example, I once worked with a gentleman who began having deception indicated on his polygraphs after a history of passing them. The polygrapher let us know that he was coming up deceptive, specifically on the question asking if he had gone out of the county without permission. This individual was pretty obsessive about things, and he had a map on which he had outlined all the county lines in our area and laid out all the routes he took to various places. He was insistent that he was not leaving the county. It took a bit to figure out, but it turns out that while it was true that he was not leaving the county, he was going to a local clothing-optional beach. He was aware that his probation officer would not have permitted him to be there, and shortly before he failed the polygraph, he had seen a child there. It is designated as an eighteen and up area, but another person brought their child, and the child and my client saw each other. The client's original crime was exposing himself to children, so he was well aware that having a child see him without his clothes on would be a significant issue for his treatment providers and probation officer. So even though the polygraph question did not ask about the nude beach, it brought to his mind something about places he was going to that he was being deceptive about. He had a deceptive result on the exam though technically, he was telling the truth as he had not gone out of the county.

Treatment providers, judges, and probation/parole officers need to remember that we do not always know why someone had a deception-indicated result on a polygraph, and further discussion is always important.

Earlier, I mentioned four polygraph exams, so let's talk about each one, how they are used, and how to prepare clients. Every treatment program is a bit different and may use polygraphs differently, so what I'm describing may vary a bit. Appropriately preparing clients for polygraph exams is an important component of good quality ethical treatment.

1. Instant Offense Polygraph

This polygraph is specifically about the offense for which the individual is on probation. This exam focuses on that specific offense and whether or not the individual has been truthful about what happened. It is not unusual for there to be details or assertions in the police report that the client tells us are not accurate or behaviors that the client tells us that they did engage in that are not reflected in the police report or victim statements. This polygraph helps sort out what happened. Knowing what behavior the client engaged in helps ensure that they are receiving the appropriate treatment and also that they are being honest, which is an important component of treatment success. Clients typically sit for this type of polygraph in our program after completing phase one of treatment. Some providers I am aware of have clients sit for this polygraph within the first few weeks of starting treatment. However, I have found that this can set clients up for failure. It is challenging to be honest about behavior you are ashamed about and have just gotten into big trouble for. This is especially true when you have just started treatment and have not had a chance to get to know your therapist or probation officer yet or have had a chance to settle in and get used to the requirements of treatment and probation. Having some time to get to know their providers and get used to what treatment and probation are like helps clients relax, and usually, they are much more honest after a few months than they are after a few weeks. There are, of course, exceptions to that rule. Sometimes clients insist that they did not commit the offense they are in trouble for. They often report that they agreed to a deal in court based on the advice of their lawyer and parents but that, in actuality, they did not commit the crime. Usually, we give those youth a little while to settle in and get to know us, but if they are still sticking to their story, we will do an instant offense polygraph sooner rather than later. It is not ethical or useful to treat someone for a problem they do not have. No ethical doctor would take out the appendix of someone with a healthy appendix.

Similarly, sex offense-specific treatment is only appropriate for someone with a sexual behavior problem. The treatment goals would be very different if a client truly appears not to have engaged in inappropriate sexual behavior. Most clients who are court-ordered to treatment do have a sexual behavior problem. However, now and again, we work with someone who did not commit the crime they are in trouble for. Polygraph exams are a useful way to help make sure we can identify clients who truly do not need the treatment.

The instant offense polygraph is usually done within the first six months of treatment. The treatment provider must ensure that they have established a good therapeutic relationship with the client. No one wants to be totally honest about things that make them feel vulnerable when they do not have a good relationship with the person they are talking to. Preparation for the instant offense polygraph should include discussing the client's thinking before the offense. For example, it is important for a client to identify their thoughts before the offense, both about why they should not engage in that behavior and how they convinced themselves it was okay to do it anyway. Clients should discuss what grooming behaviors they engaged in and identify any bribes, tricks, threats, or force used. As they work on identifying and talking through their thinking before the offense, they can use that to start writing out a complete offense description. The description should include but is not limited to a description of how they know the person they victimized and what type of relationship they had with that person. They should also discuss how much contact they had with the person prior to, during, and after the abuse. They should identify any bribes, tricks, manipulation, and/or force used and describe everything they remember about the offense. In addition, they should discuss what they said and did and what the person they victimized said and did.

The client's complete offense description can be compared to the police report and other information, like victim statements. Any discrepancies can be discussed with the client. The police report and detailed offense description should be provided to the polygraph examiner so they can have the information they need to write appropriate questions for the exam.

The client should also report if they have any additional victims that are not part of the instant offense. They do not need to give a detailed description of other inappropriate/illegal behavior at this time but do need to let their treatment provider know if they have additional victims. As with all polygraphs, it is important to remember that there are many reasons one might be deceptive on an exam that may not be directly related to the specific question being asked.

In our program, if a client has a deception indicated result on an instant offense polygraph, we usually give them some time to talk that through and see if they can figure out what is going on before taking an additional instant offense exam. If they have deception indicated on two exams in a row, we will generally have them take a sexual history polygraph within a few months. The reason for encouraging the client to disclose other victims before the instant offense polygraph is that we have found that clients who are hiding additional victims will sometimes have deceptive reactions to questions about their instant offense since they know they are deceptive about other inappropriate sexual behavior—letting us know that the other behavior that happened preempts that problem from occurring. If the client continues to have a deception-indicated result after a couple of attempts, we will generally switch to one of the other types of exams to help sort out the issue. A deception-indicated result on a polygraph exam does not indicate guilt. It indicates that something is going on that needs to be figured out.

2. Sexual History Polygraph

This next type of polygraph exam is basically just what it sounds like. To prepare for this exam, clients should have a very good understanding of consent. In our treatment program, clients generally take the sexual history polygraph part through phase two, which is sometime between six and eighteen months into treatment for most youth. The preparation for the sexual history polygraph involves the client discussing all sexual experiences that they can recall. This should include what they have seen, heard, done to others or was done to them, details of any additional people they victimized, sexual contact with animals, consensual sexual activity, pornography use, and masturbation. The history should be reviewed with the client often, at least a few times, as it is easy to forget things or be too embarrassed to talk about something, and clients often need to edit this more than once. Once the client reports that they are very sure they have talked about everything, the report can go to the polygraph examiner.

Sometimes clients decide not to talk about something relevant until they are already in the pre-polygraph interview with the polygraph examiner. The goal is for the client to talk about everything with their treatment provider, not to "confess" at the last minute to the polygraph examiner. Depending on the nature of the "confession," the polygraph exam can sometimes move forward. This is usually the case if whatever the client was holding onto is relatively minor, such as admitting that they had some alcohol at a family gathering or went out of the county with their parent and did not ask or inform their probation officer. However, if the confession is more significant, for example, having additional past victims or being alone with a child, then the polygraph cannot take place, and they will have to be scheduled again at a later date after they have discussed the situation with their treatment provider. The polygraph examiner that I have been working with for many years told me once that he does that because the rush of relief or the worry about consequences that a person gets from confessing to something they have been holding back can interfere with the polygraph results and perhaps mask other things that someone might be being deceptive about.

Sometimes there are special circumstances that impact a client's polygraph exam. We already discussed that clients who report that they are innocent usually take their instant offense polygraph earlier than is typical. If the client has no deception indicated on the instant offense polygraph, they usually take a sexual history polygraph fairly soon after. That polygraph focuses specifically on checking any history of inappropriate sexual behavior. If a client has no deception indicated on that polygraph, they are usually released from treatment as they do not have a sexual behavior problem, and it is not appropriate for them to participate in that type of treatment. A few of the clients I have had in this situation remained in treatment, but the goal of treatment changed to working on their trauma, as that was a significant problem for them and the treatment they benefited from.

Another special circumstance that can impact polygraph preparation is clients who come from families with multi-generational chronic complex trauma. Many youths in our treatment program have engaged in so much sexual behavior with relatives that they cannot recall all the individual incidents or be able to think about their history in a chronological way, which is not at all unusual for individuals with trauma. Creating a detailed sexual history document is nearly impossible for these clients, and rather than setting them up for failure by having the polygraph question be something like, "Have you told your therapist about all your sexual behavior?" questions like, "Is there any sexual behavior that you are deliberately withholding (or keeping secret) from your therapist?" help make it possible for the youth to be successful and do not punish them for things that are outside their control.

Another issue that can arise is that sometimes youth are unwilling to talk about something because they are protecting a loved one. We had a client struggling with his sexual history polygraph many years ago. This client was generally well-behaved and did not have any trouble complying with probation requirements. For the most part, he was also open and honest in treatment and was overall doing well. I strongly suspected he had been abused by someone in the family, though he denied it for a long while. He was protecting an older family member, who he knew was undocumented. He was aware that I was obligated to report any abuse he had experienced since he was a minor and concerned that if he reported what had happened to him, this loved one would come to the attention of law enforcement and be deported. He was unwilling to take the risk that his loved one would be harmed, even if it meant risking his own success. Luckily the situation resolved well, and his loved one did not have any immigration issues, and my client was able to get the help he needed without feeling like he was risking harm to his family. That is an example of the importance of looking at the whole picture, not just relying on the results of one assessment tool. We knew from the polygraph that he was being deceptive about something, but we also knew from knowing him that it was not likely to be something that was causing harm to anyone and that, given enough time and space, he would let us know what was going on.

Some clients will need more extensive and comprehensive treatment than other clients need. One of the factors we use to determine if a client would benefit from a briefer course of treatment is how they handle the polygraph exams. In general, if a client can have a no deception indicated result on both the instant offense and sexual history polygraph exams the first time they take them with no significant admissions, they are put on what we call the "honesty track." When we started doing this, we called it the fast track, but some clients still chose to take a very long time to do the smaller work, and the name confused the court. Clients on the honesty track are asked to complete phase one of treatment, giving them a basic overview of all the treatment concepts, but they are only expected to complete all four phases of a few chapters rather than the full program. For most clients on the honesty track, those four chapters in the workbook we use are "Rules," "Escaping Risk," "Positive Sexuality," and "Impulse Control". However, the specific chapters sometimes change depending on the client's individual needs. Part of the role of the polygrapher on the treatment team is to help ensure that the treatment plan is individualized to the client's specific needs, which is one of the ways in which that happens.

3. Maintenance Polygraph

The third type of polygraph exam focuses on whether the client is being honest about what probation rules they have broken. In our program, this type of polygraph is usually given to clients when there is reason to believe they may be engaging in behavior that they are not being honest about. For example, sometimes a client may not attend school or stay out past curfew, and the parents do not know what the child is doing or where they are. Maintenance polygraphs can help sort out what is going on with that youth.

4. Monitoring Polygraph

The fourth type of polygraph looks at the question of whether the youth has reoffended. This exam is generally given to clients who have either been alone with a child or who have had deception indicated on multiple sexual history polygraphs. In some instances, a specific issue examination may have to be administered if a client has either been accused of a specific crime or is alleged to have a new victim. A specific issue test is usually the most accurate type of exam in those circumstances. This type of exam is very helpful for clients who might get accused of behavior they are not engaging in. For example, I remember an adult client who struggled with someone in the community who knew he was on probation and would call the probation office to report that they had seen this client with children or doing something else he was not supposed to be doing. When this first started happening, the client was extremely worried that he would be incarcerated since the things he was being accused of were major violations of his probation rules, but a polygraph helped establish that the accusations were untrue and just a reflection of that particular community member's long-standing dislike of my client's family.

While they are controversial, I have found that polygraph exams are a useful part of a comprehensive treatment program when used as a treatment tool and administered by a qualified high-quality polygrapher. As I said earlier, there is not a lot of research to look at about using polygraphs with people in treatment, but there is at least one study that showed that clients tended to disclose significantly more victims when in a treatment program that uses polygraph exams (Harrison and Eliot, 1999). When clients disclose previously unknown victims, those children can be identified, and the adults in their lives can get them help. An important component of sex offense-specific treatment is community safety and prevention. Ensuring that more victims of sexual trauma get access to the help they need is one of the ways to do that. Clients are often concerned that they will get into more legal trouble if they admit to additional victims. I have never had a client get into any additional legal trouble for something they did before being placed on probation that they admitted to during their treatment. Judges and district attorneys are typically aware that being honest in treatment is a good sign. Lawyers have told me that clients have protection under the Fifth Amendment against self-incrimination since the polygraph exams are part of court-ordered treatment. It is important to remember that a polygraph is a treatment tool, so if an additional pending court case or issue has not yet been adjudicated, a polygraph done as part of the treatment would not be ethically appropriate.

Chapter 6

Families of Youth in Treatment

Working with youth generally means working with their adult family members. Sometimes that can be the most challenging part of working with youth. Before I went back to school for my master's degree, I was a preschool teacher for a little while, and while spending all day in a room full of one-year-olds was tiring, dealing with the other adults at the preschool was one of the reasons I only worked there for a relatively short time. Families of children in legal trouble for their sexual behavior are usually under enormous stress. From the moment the behavior comes to light, parents have to navigate the Child Protective Services system, the legal system, the reactions of other people in their lives, and then the requirements of both treatment and probation. Some families have more emotional and financial resources than others, but it is stressful and overwhelming for all of them.

When juveniles offend sexually, the person they victimized is usually someone they are close to and have easy access to, so often it is another family member. While that is not always the case, parents are typically trying to help both the child who committed the offense and the child who was victimized. If the victimized child is a niece, nephew, cousin, stepchild, or family friend, then parents also have to manage the relationships with other adults in the family who may be reacting to the situation in ways that are very different from their own. For some families, the information about the sexual behavior problem can change custody agreements and impact visitation schedules.

Sexual behavior problems and sexual trauma are also often multigenerational. It is not unusual for some of the adults involved to have had their own experiences with being abused. Dealing with what their child did can bring up their own unresolved trauma and be overwhelming. No matter why the child is in therapy, parents with children in therapy often worry about being judged, and parents of youth who sexually offend are impacted by that worry as well. Especially in the beginning, it can sometimes be hard for parents to feel comfortable with the treatment providers as they are concerned with defending their child and their own parenting. Often, especially since the child typically has more frequent and regular contact with the treatment provider than the parents do, the child is quicker to develop a good working relationship with their therapist than the parents are.

For many reasons, parents are usually overwhelmed and very nervous when meeting the treatment providers for the first time. The families must understand what to expect in treatment, how forensic work differs from bringing their child to a therapist voluntarily, what is expected of their child, and what is expected of them.

In our program, we have the family orientation handbook given to the family at the initial intake session. This handbook covers all the information about how treatment works, what to expect, what is expected of them, the risks and rewards of treatment, and information about how they can be successful. We ask that families take this book home, read it aloud together, write down any questions they have, and then schedule their next meeting to discuss it. This book helps give families the information they need and serves as an informed consent document. Since it is a printed book, it gives families information they can easily refer back to later. When a child starts treatment, they have often just gone through the court system, met their probation officer, and been ordered to begin treatment. They are usually overwhelmed and extremely nervous, so it is sometimes difficult for them to retain information from their first appointment or think about what questions they have. Having a written handbook that they can go back to and reread, which encourages them to write down and ask questions, helps ensure that they truly understand what treatment is like and what is being asked of them and of their child.

When a family starts treatment, one of the first questions is, "How long is this going to take?" We let them know the average time that youth spend in treatment and that the answer to that question depends mostly on what the client does in treatment and their individual needs. We also let them know that we have seen that those youth whose families are involved and supportive usually move through the program more quickly, and those youth who do not have family support usually take longer.

Parents of youth in our program are expected to go through chaperone training and attend monthly parent groups, though groups have been put on hold due to pandemic safety. We also ask that parents help remind their youth to do their treatment work, though, for some parents, we have to be clear that they are not supposed to do their youth's work for them. Just remind them to do their own work. Parents must be aware that they are not responsible for "making" the youth do the work. It is also helpful if parents support and help enforce treatment and probation rules. Most parents do their best to help their youth succeed, but that is not always the case. Despite court orders and therapy recommendations, we have worked with youth whose adults leave them in charge of younger children, sometimes even leaving them alone with the child they previously victimized. Sometimes families will take their child out of town without getting permission from their probation officer, and sometimes they will take the youth to places not considered appropriate. We have families bring youth to child-centered places—theme parks, elementary school Halloween carnivals—without a safety plan and to places more adult-orientated. I'll never forget the first time a young teenager in the program had parents who took him to dinner at Hooters for his birthday. I thought it was an odd place to bring your middle schooler for his birthday, especially if said middle schooler is already on probation for inappropriate sexual behavior. However, since that first family, it has happened more than once with other families in our program, so I'm no longer surprised. I often use that as an example when talking to parents about what might not be a good idea to do while their child is on probation.

While some parents are unwilling or unable to enforce rules like curfew or travel restrictions, leaving their children to manage the many treatment and probation requirements on their own, some families have the opposite struggle. While not as common as families who will not or cannot develop enough stability to support their children, some families are so controlling and strict that their youth do not get a chance to practice making choices and evaluating the safety and risk levels of situations on their own.

We had a family concerned about possible stigma or consequences for their son at school once the offense came to light, so they decided to homeschool. While at home for school, this young man was not even allowed to decide when he needed to go to the bathroom or get water or food, as he could only get up from his computer at the scheduled times his father had decided upon. This family would also not allow this young man to get a job as they did not want him to cross a busy street by himself to get to the neighborhood where there were stores he could work at. This was a very smart older teenager who could figure out when to go to the bathroom and how to walk through a neighborhood safely. These parents were very concerned that their son was immature and asked me more than once to help him work on behaving like an adult, but actively did things that kept him from engaging in adult life skills. Not surprisingly, when he went to college the next year, he struggled as he had no experience making decisions.

Parenting under any circumstance is about finding the balance between providing help and support and not controlling or smothering so that youth can try out new things and figure out how to make safe, healthy decisions. That is true for all youth, but in many ways, particularly when a child has already engaged in significantly inappropriate and illegal behavior and needs to practice good decision-making skills. It is a difficult balance to achieve. It is helpful for parents to develop good working relationships with the treatment providers to have a collaborative team approach.

There is a chapter on chaperone training later in the book, so I will not go into it in great detail here. In brief, chaperone training is designed to give adults the information they need to help safely supervise a person who has committed a sex offense when they are around younger children. The adults are not responsible for the child's behavior; the child is responsible for their behavior, but adults are responsible for providing good structure and supervision.

Before the pandemic crisis, our program had chaperone training sessions as a group that met for several hours an afternoon or two on the weekends. During the pandemic crisis, we had no groups, so chaperone training has been happening individually in telehealth sessions. The number of sessions varies from client to client, but four to six sessions are typical. The content of chaperone training is specific to youth in the treatment program, but I am often contacted by families or Child Protective Services about situations that involve children who have acted out sexually but have not been prosecuted or court-ordered to treatment. Families and caseworkers often want guidelines and advice about keeping everyone safe moving forward. Chaperone information can be modified for the individual family and situation. However, it is more difficult to predict what problems may arise when working with a family whose child is not in treatment.

Another requirement of treatment is monthly parent groups. Those have been on hold during the pandemic but will likely resume once it is safe. We ask that every child in treatment have at least one adult that comes to the parent group; it is helpful if it is usually the same adult for consistency, but that is not always the case. It is not limited to one adult. Often, both parents, stepparents, and other involved family members come. The group has several benefits for the parents who attend. In general, youth with parents who take treatment and probation seriously are more likely to take them seriously themselves, and they generally move through the program faster. Parents who attend the group regularly show their youth that they take that commitment seriously. The parent group serves as a support group for the parents. Having a child on probation for committing a sex offense can be a very isolating experience. Many families choose not to share that information with most people in their lives, and as a result, they can feel isolated and alone. Sometimes the offense itself creates a rift in the family, and parents find themselves no longer talking to close friends and family members who used to be a source of support.

Meeting with other parents in the same situation helps parents realize that they are not alone, that other families are successfully navigating this, and that they can too. Generally, in a group, there are parents of youth who have just started treatment, youth who have been in treatment for a little while, and youth who are almost done. New parents benefit from talking to parents who have already figured out how to manage probation and treatment requirements, and seeing that clients successfully graduate from treatment and are released from probation is a source of hope when it seems like the process might be endless. The new parents remind adults whose children have been in treatment for a while of how they used to feel and can see how far their youth have come and how far they have come as a family. Parent groups are also a good source of information. Each month, we use the time to explain one of the workbook chapters, so parents have a better idea of what their children are learning, why, and their typical struggles with each concept. In addition, it is a good place for parents to ask any questions and express any concerns. While we occasionally have had a group of parents who sit quietly and do not ask questions or engage in conversation, parents usually end up enjoying their time chatting with each other and sharing experiences.

Chapter 7

Chaperone Training

I t is important to remember that being on probation or in treatment does not suddenly transform children and adolescents into little adults. They are still youth going through the same developmental milestones and have the same needs and desires as other youth. Some treatment programs insist on limiting the youth's ability to do almost everything typical of other youth their age. While some limits are unavoidable, especially in inpatient settings, there are many things youth on probation can and should safely do, including socializing, getting a job, extracurricular activities at school, and masturbation. What these children need for healthy development is not any different from what other youth their age need. The desired result is for youth in treatment to become healthy, well-functioning adults in the future, so it makes sense to help them learn how to navigate typical teenage experiences safely and healthily.

Keeping a child isolated from peers and unable to participate in family or school activities does not allow for healthy development. We cannot expect children to grow into healthy, functioning adults if we do not allow them the necessary experiences. We also cannot expect them to learn how to evaluate risk levels and make good choices if they never get the chance to practice. Of course, keeping the community safe is one of the top priorities of treatment and probation. It is also not appropriate to simply throw youth into what may be high-risk situations without any knowledge, support, or monitoring. The key is finding a good balance, allowing clients to have the developmental experiences typical for people their age while also putting structure and boundaries in place that allow those things to happen safely.

Many components go into deciding what is and what is not okay for an individual client to be involved in. Typically youth get more privileges as time goes on, and they have shown a willingness to be safe and demonstrated knowledge of treatment concepts. In addition, probation officers and treatment providers evaluate the specifics of individual events, for example sleeping over at a same-age friend's house who has no younger siblings versus a friend who has younger siblings; or a typical school field trip versus a youth I worked with once who was taking a child development class and was supposed to go on a field trip to a preschool to help teach for a day. It is important to look at each adolescent and family for the individuals they are and each event or trip for the specific issues that might come up.

Chaperone training is one component that helps ensure safety in the home and at family gatherings and other activities. Chaperone training is offered to the adults who will be supervising the child when they are around younger children. Typically, the child's parents participate, and other adults like aunts, uncles, adult siblings, and grandparents involved with the child will also participate. Chaperones are given a training manual and participate in some training sessions. Before the pandemic, the training was usually done in a group setting. For safety reasons, it has now moved to individual sessions. Group chaperone training allows parents to hear each other's questions and concerns, so that is an advantage. Individual chaperone training allows families to get training shortly after their child starts the treatment program, rather than waiting until we have enough parents to form a group. That is an advantage of that format.

The role of a chaperone is to be present when the child with sexual behavior problems is around children who are more than two years younger than them. The presence of the chaperone helps provide a barrier to the child reoffending and protection from the child being accused of reoffending when they did not. Often abuse happens between family members, and sometimes the families will choose to go through the reunification process, so in cases where the child who committed the offense and the child (or children) who were victimized are siblings, it may be that they eventually will both be living in the same household again. Usually, when the abuse has happened between siblings, the child who engaged in the abuse is removed from the household for a time, often living with other relatives if they are in outpatient treatment or sometimes living at an inpatient treatment facility. Sometimes, however, the judge will allow the family to continue living together without any separation period. The specifics of how families can safely live together will vary from family to family, but chaperone training is an important component. Even if the child who committed the sex offense has no younger siblings and will not be living with the person they victimized, their adults need to understand how to supervise them safely and what to be mindful of when they are around younger children.

Chaperone training is a place to get information and for the adults to ask questions. We usually start by asking the adults to give us a list of questions or topics they would like to see covered in training to ensure that all of their concerns are addressed. Prior to taking chaperone training, families in our program have all been provided with the family orientation handbook. Typically the child has already started working with their treatment provider, and both the child and their adults have gotten a feel for how probation and treatment work. The chaperone training is another opportunity to make sure the adults understand what to expect and how to support their children. In addition to having a chaperone with them when appropriate, youth on probation can also write safety plans to be able to go on trips or to events that would typically not be allowed for someone who is on probation.

It is sometimes difficult for parents to figure out when a child needs to complete a safety plan and/or have their chaperone with them and when they do not. Determining that is a good illustration of how working as a treatment team is useful. A probation officer's role is to determine where someone on probation is allowed or not allowed to go. There are also treatment issues to take into consideration for some events.

In our program, youth are asked to first check in with their probation officer about an upcoming trip or event that they would like to attend. Once their officer tells them that it will be okay with a safety plan, the child then writes a safety plan and presents it to their treatment provider for approval. Once the safety plan is approved, they can then show it to their probation officer, allowing everyone to be on the same page about what will happen. For a safety plan to be useful, the client must have a pretty detailed understanding of what will happen on the trip. For example, suppose a family plans to go out of town over the weekend. In that case, the client needs to know where they are going, what the sleeping venue and arrangements will be, and have some idea of what activities they might be participating in.

Often youth will try to present safety plans for trips or events without knowledge of what will happen. Sometimes, that is because the family has not decided yet, and sometimes it is because the adolescent forgot to ask or forgot what their parent told them. Occasionally it is because the child does not really want to go on the trip, and rather than just telling their parent that, they try to do a bad job on the assignment so they can tell their parents that we told them they could not go. Some families tend to be more spontaneous in their plans, and it can be a big adjustment for them to get used to going through the approval process to do things, making spontaneity all but impossible.

Some families have a particular trip or event that is pretty repetitive. For example, a child might write a safety plan for going to the pool at their apartment complex. We would not ask them to write a separate plan and get it approved every time they go to the pool, and we generally have them write one good quality safety plan and use that every time. Similarly, we had a youth in the treatment program who had older relatives who lived in a town several hours away. It was very common for this family to visit with the extended family on the weekends, and they went there at least every month or two. The trip itself, the people who were going to be there, and the activities involved (barbecue, dominoes, and hanging out, if I remember correctly) were always the same. Rather than go through the whole approval process every time, this client wrote a safety plan that included all the relevant information, and his probation officer told him that he needed to call and leave a voicemail every time they went to let the probation officer know what dates they would be gone. Once that was in place, the family could go back and forth to the relatives' house without having to do a lot of upfront planning. The client also knew that if something was significantly different about a particular trip there—different sleeping arrangements or young children visiting—they would need to let everyone know and adjust their safety plan accordingly. The same approach can work for safety plans for events. For example, if the child has a field trip to an amusement or water park, they will need an individual safety plan. However, if the child is in the band or on the football team, they will not need an individual safety plan for every game. They will likely just write a general safety plan for home games and a general safety plan for away games and then be able to participate in their activities without worrying about remembering to get approval in time for every event.

A chaperone can be defined as a person who accompanies and looks after a person or group of people. If the client is attending a trip or event with no increased risk, for example, they will be with adults and all the youth going are their age or older, there may not be a need for the chaperone to be involved. If, however, the situation involves greater risk, for example, a family gathering where there will be younger children, it is important for an adult who knows the child's history of sexual behavior problems and has gone through chaperone training to be there. This helps keep everyone safe, including the client. Over the years, we have had youth in the program be accused of additional inappropriate behavior by someone when they had not engaged in that behavior. Chaperones help protect the youth from reoffending and help protect them from being accused of reoffending.

In our program, we use a chaperone treatment manual specific to the content and style of our treatment manual, so parents get information that fits in with and complements the knowledge they acquired when their child started treatment. Often I am asked to deliver chaperone training to families who do not have a child on probation but have a child who has caused concern for the adults in their lives. Chaperone training can certainly be adjusted for a particular family's needs. Still, it is more complex and less effective when the adults do not have the base understanding of treatment concepts that comes with having youth in treatment. The treatment provider does not know the individual child and family well enough to have a good idea of what particular issues might be the most important for them.

In general, chaperone training addresses several topics, including but not limited to: defining and discussing the role and responsibilities of a chaperone, talking about rules, risk, and safety plans, talking about how and why sex offenses happen, information about thinking errors, discussing myths and facts about youth with sexual behavior problems, and going over signs that might indicate a child is returning to a problematic pattern of behavior or is being abused. In addition, there is information about child development, parenting, and common characteristics of youth in treatment.

Chapter 8

Clarification and Reunification

Most sexual abuses happen between people who know each other. That is true for adults who commit sex crimes and true for juveniles. The person who was victimized is often a relative, typically a sibling or a cousin, or perhaps a close family friend. When the behavior initially comes to light, and the children live in the same house, the child who offended is typically, though not always, removed from the home. That can be very difficult for families. If the parents were already living separately, they might be able to alternate visitation and custody schedules so the children are not in the same household at the same time. In families where the parents live together, or only one parent is available, the child who has offended is sometimes taken in by other relatives and stays with grandparents, aunts, uncles, or close family friends. Sometimes the parents can get a second dwelling, and one parent moves with one of the children into a separate home or apartment, which is also stressful and not typically sustainable for long periods.

It is common for part of the pre-court and probation conditions for the child in legal trouble to require that they have no contact with the person they victimized until approved by treatment providers and the court. Some families can reunify reasonably quickly, and I have worked with cases in which the judge decided not to have the child who offended move out at all, so there was no separation. However, for many families, this period of separation can last a long time and put a great deal of emotional and financial strain on them. Generally, once the inappropriate or illegal behavior is identified, the children are separated, often by their parents at first and later by Child Protective Services or court order. There is a period of assessment and treatment, then clarification and apology, followed by reunification. While it is common for children who are in trouble for their sexual behavior to be court-ordered to treatment, children who were victimized are not usually subject to a court order about treatment. However, for clarification and reunification to occur, it is imperative that both children have an appropriate treatment provider.

It is not unusual for the adults in the family to let us know that reunification is a major goal and one of their top priorities. Sometimes that process goes fairly smoothly and relatively quickly, though rarely as quickly as the family would like. Sometimes, however, the process can take a long time. There are a lot of factors involved in clarification and reunification. While it is the best option for the vast majority of families, it is not the best option for everyone, and sometimes it is not something that happens at all, no matter how much the adults in the family want it.

Before clarification or reunification can happen, it is important to ensure everyone is ready and that everyone involved will benefit from the process, and no one will be harmed. The child in treatment for their sexual behavior problems will hopefully be working through assignments related to clarification and reunification, and the process cannot begin until they are in a place to be helpful to the child they victimized. The child who was victimized must have a therapist of their own. Nothing should move forward until the therapist working with the victimized child believes the process will benefit the client.

Most children who have been victimized by a sibling I have worked with want to reunify and are often annoyed and frustrated that the process is taking longer than they would like, but that is not always the case. In cases where I have been the victimized child's therapist, I have sometimes been told by the adults that the child does want to see the older sibling, only to find out from the child that that is the last thing they want to have happen and that the idea is extremely bothersome. Sometimes even when the sibling who was victimized does want to reunify, there are aspects of the process that are stressful for them for one reason or another. The therapist working with the victimized child must communicate with the treatment team so that the process can be immediately slowed down or paused if there is any stress or problems for that child. The victimized child is the person who determines most aspects of how clarification and reunification are going to go. Their well-being is the guiding factor in making decisions about contact.

So how does one figure out when the various people involved are ready to move forward with clarification and reunification? For the person who was victimized, typically positive signs include that they can talk about and tolerate conversations about the abuse, their trauma symptoms have diminished, they can self-regulate enough to handle conversations that may cause big feelings, they want the contact to occur, and they feel safe enough that contact is not detrimental or problematic for them. For the child who offended, positive signs include:

- Acknowledging that the abuse happened
- Comprehending the impact their behavior had on others
- Recognizing the need to change their behavior in order to keep people safe
- Willingness to consider the needs and feelings of their sibling
- Learning and employing the ability to self-regulate and manage their own emotional reaction to conversations about the abuse
- Willingness to follow treatment and family safety rules

In addition to the children involved, the adults must be ready to handle the process. Positive signs that the adults are ready include a willingness to acknowledge that the abusive behavior took place, a willingness to place responsibility for that behavior appropriately, the ability to support all the children, the ability to manage their own emotional responses to conversations about the abuse, and a willingness to follow safety recommendations.

Often, the victimized child is ready to reunify before the child who offended is. The child who offended must be able and willing to take responsibility for their behavior and acknowledge the harm that was caused. It is not unusual for the child who offended to struggle with fully acknowledging the harm they caused because of their own shame, and getting to the point where they can be helpful to the person they hurt can sometimes take a while.

Our program usually has clients write two letters: a clarification letter and an apology letter. The purpose of the clarification letter is to clarify to the person who was victimized that the abuse was entirely the responsibility of the person who abused them and that they did nothing wrong and did not cause the abuse to happen to them. In this letter, the child who offended also discusses some of the harm they have caused and how that may have made the victimized child feel. This letter can be very difficult to write and takes a great deal of time, reflection, and work on the part of the child in treatment. The letter has a lot of required components, and the language must be carefully crafted to ensure that it does not contain thinking errors and that it is age-appropriate for whatever age the victimized child is at the time. We do not have clients apologize in this letter or ask for forgiveness, as we do not want the victimized child to feel any pressure to say "That's okay" or to tell the person they forgive them. Once the clarification process has begun, the child in treatment can present a second letter called the apology letter. In the apology letter, the child who has offended can talk about their dedication to being safe and responsible, and they can tell the person they victimized that they are sorry. If they want, they can ask for forgiveness.

The specific content of the clarification letter varies as the details are specific to the individual involved, but the format is fairly similar. Different treatment workbooks have different instructions for clarification letters, though most of the workbooks I have used have similar approaches and instructions. Here are the instructions from a treatment book called *Beacon*, written by Nicolas Carrasco, which I most often use with clients. The following instructions for writing a clarification letter are based on teachings from Timothy J. Kahn in his book *Pathways*.

Writing the Clarification Letter

A clarification letter does just what the name says. It "clarifies" or "makes clear" for the victim what happened during the abuse. It talks about before, during, and after the abuse, and it helps to make clear to the victim that the abuse was **not** their fault. It makes clear that you are responsible for the abuse. It also explains to your victim that they are a good person and did the right in telling about the abuse.

This assignment will take a long time; you will have to redo it several times. If you have a computer, write it on the computer. Be sure to keep a copy of all the different versions you do. In writing your letter, follow the guidelines below. Some guidelines tell you what to do, and some tell you what not to do. In this entire letter, you must be very careful with your words. The most important thing is that you do not hurt the victim by what you say to them, and how you say things does not blame the victim.

- **The tone of the letter should be serious.**

What NOT to say:

✗　*Dear Joe, WUZ UP!!!!!*

Example of what to say:

✔　*Dear Joe,*

- **Do not make statements that sound like you are trying to manipulate the victim or trying to make them feel sorry for you.**

> What NOT to say:
>
> ✗ *I really missed you.*
> *I am really sorry I hurt you.*
> *I really hope you will read this letter.*
>
> Example of what to say:
>
> ✓ *Thank you for agreeing to read/listen to this letter.*

- **Do not tell the victim what they should think, feel, or do.**

> What NOT to say:
>
> ✗ *I don't want you to feel …*
> *Don't think that…*
> *You can…*
>
> Example of what to say:
>
> ✓ *I'm not sure how you feel, but you may have felt . . .*

Sentences like these show that you are still trying to control the victim or trying to tell the victim what to do.

- **Do not ask questions.** Most of us start a letter by asking questions like, *"How are you doing?"* or *"How's it going?"* Don't do that in this case. I recommend starting the letter by thanking the victim for accepting the letter. For example,

---

What NOT to say:

✗ *How are you doing?*

Example of what to say:

✔ *Thank you for accepting my letter.*
Thank you for agreeing to read/listen to my letter.

- **Let the victim know that they can decide whether to read this letter.** The purpose of this is so that the victim will feel like they have control, something that they did not have during the abuse, but again be careful not to tell the victim what they should think, feel, or do.

What NOT to say:

✗ *Tell me if you want to hear this letter or not.*

Example of what to say:

✔ *You are very brave for agreeing to read/listen to this letter. However, it might be painful. If at any time it becomes too hard to read/listen to, you can tell me to stop, and I will.*

- **Explain to the victim how you abused them, but do it so that the victim does not feel abused again.** In this section of the letter, include your grooming behaviors.

> What NOT to say:
>
> ✗ *That time that I [very graphic examples of the abuse].*
>
> Example of what to say:
>
> ✓ *I let you play with my video game all the time before I touched you. You thought I was being nice to you, but that was my way of tricking you so that I could hurt you later on.*
>
> *I told you Mom would hit us if you told her that I was touching you. That was a way of tricking you so that you would not tell and so I would not get caught.*

- **Explain to the victim that they were in no way responsible for the abuse. Make a clear statement that YOU are responsible for having hurt them.**

> What NOT to say:
>
> ✗ *It was my fault, BUT you shouldn't have come into my room. If YOU hadn't come into my room . . .*
>
> Example of what to say:
>
> ✓ *You did nothing wrong. The abuse was entirely because of the choices I made.*

- **Explain how you used their good qualities to abuse them.**

> What NOT to say:
>
> ✗ *You are a trusting person, and that's why I was able to hurt you.*
>
> Using the example from earlier, you might say:
>
> ✓ *You are a very trusting person. When I let you play my video games all the time, you trusted me, thinking that I was being a nice person and that I was not going to hurt you. Trust is a good thing to have, and you were right to trust me. It was me who was wrong by using the trust you had in me to hurt you.*

- **Explain to the victim in words they might understand how the abuse hurt them and how it might hurt them in the future.**

> What NOT to say:
>
> ✗ *I know exactly how you are feeling.*
>
> It is important to say that you do not know exactly how they felt or might feel now. You might say something like:
>
> ✓ *I don't know exactly how you feel, but I am sure that I hurt you in many ways. Some of the ways I think I hurt you are:*
>
> ✓ You can also say:
> *I also know that I hurt your family. I think I might have hurt them in these ways. I hurt your parents …*
> *I hurt your brother/sister …*

✔ You can also talk about how he/she will continue to be hurt in the future by saying something like:

I think that in the future, you will think about how I hurt you when...

In the future, your parents will be reminded about how I hurt you when...

In the future, your parents might...

- **Make a sincere (really says what you think and feel) closing statement and offer to answer any questions that they might have.**

What NOT to say:

✗ *I wrote this so you would know everything and it should have all the information you need about what happened, so now you should understand.*

Example of what to say:

✔ *I hope what I have written will help you in understanding what happened and in knowing that none of what happened was your fault. All the hurt was caused by me and not by you. I would like to let you know that if you have any questions, I am willing to answer anything you might ask.*

CLARIFICATION LETTER EXAMPLE

Dear [name of the child who was victimized],

Thank you for reading/listening to this letter. I am writing this letter to let you know that it is not your fault that I hurt you, and all the painful things that I did to you were because of decisions I made, not because of anything that you did. Also, in this letter, I will explain how I hurt you and how I think that what I did affected you.

You are very brave for agreeing to read/listen to this letter. However, it might be painful. If at any time it becomes too hard to read/listen to, you can tell me to stop, and I will.

Whenever you got scared, I would let you enter my room. I would also listen to you about what was going on in your life. This was how I tricked you into trusting me so that I could hurt you. You did not do anything wrong, and I'm the one that was wrong. One of the things that I did was spend a lot of my time with you and let you play with my toys and games before I hurt you. It is not your fault that I took advantage of you like that, and I should not have done that. You are a loving and trusting person. Being loving and trusting are good things, and I was wrong to take advantage of that. You are also brave. I threatened to get you in trouble with Mom if you told, but you were very brave and told people what was happening anyway. Your honesty allowed you to be protected and me to get the help I needed so that I would not hurt you or anyone else again.

I do not know for sure what you have been feeling, but I can guess some of what you might be feeling. You might have wondered if this was your fault and be feeling guilty about it. This was not your fault at all. I'm the one who hurt you, and I'm really glad you told what happened. I also think I might have hurt your relationships with our parents by telling you to hide the fact that I was doing harmful things to you. I shouldn't have told you to keep secrets. Talking to Mom and Dad is a good thing. In the future, you might worry about someone hurting you again or feel it is hard to trust people. I took advantage of your trust, but it was wrong for me to do that, and it wasn't because of anything you did. If you are ever scared or uncomfortable around me, you can tell me, and I'll walk away if you do not want to tell me. You can tell Mom or Dad, and they'll let me know to go somewhere else.

I hope this helps you know what happened and why I hurt you was not your fault at all. If you have any questions, I am willing to answer them.

Typically once everyone is ready, there will be a clarification meeting. If possible, this meeting should happen in the office of the victimized child's therapist so that they are somewhere they feel safe and comfortable. Participants in that meeting usually include the victimized child, their therapist and support people the victimized child has asked for (usually parents), and the child who offended and their therapist. Depending on the family's specific needs, the child who offended will usually read the clarification letter they wrote out loud during the session. Sometimes the child who has been victimized wants to be able to preview the letter or does not want it read during the session at all. In those cases, the letter will have been sent to their therapist beforehand to review it during their therapy sessions in a time and space that is comfortable for them. Sometimes the victimized child is more comfortable exchanging letters before having an in-person meeting. In that case, they can write a letter asking questions or talking about whatever they would like and have their therapist pass that on to the offender child's therapist to go over and answer during their sessions.

A while ago, I was working with a family where the older sibling (let's call them Morgan) had abused the younger one (let's call them Finn). When the abuse came to light, Morgan was removed from the home and moved in with their grandparents. Initially, Finn was very glad to have Morgan out of the house and feel safe, both youths were in treatment, and the family did a good job of supporting both of them. It was not very long before Finn was ready to see Morgan again, though Morgan was not yet ready. Finn found the delay frustrating, and not having contact with their older sibling started impacting their mental health. Luckily Finn's therapist and I were in touch, and he let me know what was happening. Finn was able to write letters that the therapist passed on to me. Most of the letters focused on things like asking what video games Morgan was playing and what they might play together when they got the chance again, sprinkled with questions about why Morgan was not doing treatment faster so they could see each other again and how they could make sure things were safe. Morgan and I were able to go through the letters during Morgan's sessions, and Morgan got to have some time to write their responses. The exchange of letters helped Finn feel more in control and less isolated by the process and gave Morgan more time to process their own guilt and shame and think about what kind of older sibling they wanted to be. This family was able to have a successful clarification and reunification process.

Sometimes, after the initial clarification/reunification session, there are further sessions involving both therapists, and sometimes there are not. The number of sessions required depends a lot on the specifics of the individual involved and how the child who was victimized feels. After the initial session, the victimized child has at least one session with their therapist to process what happened. We then decide if we are going to have additional sessions or start moving toward allowing the family to meet on their own. Typically, when they start meeting on their own, they start with a short meeting. For example, they all go out for lunch and spend an hour or two together. Over time, the length of time that the family spends together increases. If living together in the same house is the goal, the family can eventually move to have overnight visits, then weekend visits, and then ultimately, the child with sexual behavior problems can move back home. After every contact that the victimized child and the offender child have, the victimized child must meet with their therapist, especially before making any decisions about increasing the length or frequency of contact. Sometimes this process is very smooth, and sometimes it needs to be paused or stopped for one reason or another.

The reunification process for Morgan and Finn, as mentioned earlier, went smoothly. The family easily transitioned from brief visits to longer visits, overnights, long weekends, and then moving in together. The process went slower than Finn wanted, but there was never a time when Finn or their therapist reported any distress or problems other than frustration about how long it took.

On the other hand, I remember a family moving through their reunification process and having more setbacks and delays. In that case, I was the therapist for the victimized child. The beginning of the process went pretty well, and my client was very eager to have contact with her older brother. It was a bit difficult to get the parents to follow the rules about limits on the number of times the youth saw each other and the length of time they were together, but at first, my client wasn't bothered by that. When we moved to overnight visits, the family was instructed to put an alarm on the door of the child who offended, so if he came out of his room at night when the parents were not supervising, it would go off and wake them up. The parents reported that they were doing that and were following through with setting the alarm every night. Around that time, my client, who told me everything was fine and she was happy to have her brother home more often, started acting out at home. She became defiant about chores and things that she had never been defiant about before, and she reported to me that her room was scary, and she could tell it was haunted, which was also something she had never had trouble with before. She told me that everything was fine, but her behavior indicated otherwise.

Much to the adults' frustration, we paused overnights and eventually figured out that the family had set up the alarm so that they could not hear it in the parents' bedroom, and the young man was told that when he got up in the morning, he should just turn it off, so it didn't wake anyone up. His bedroom was right next to his sister's bedroom. So they deliberately set up a situation where he was unsupervised around his sister, which was distressing for her. She hadn't initially told me that he was unsupervised, which made her nervous, as she did not want her brother to get into any more trouble and didn't want her parents to be mad at her. Once we got to the bottom of why she was having a hard time, we could return to having daytime visits only while the probation officer and the therapist for the child who had offended discussed with the parents the importance of following the required rules by probation and court.

Eventually, the parents cooperated, and reunification got back on track and got to the point where my client genuinely felt comfortable having her brother in the house again. In their desire to speed the process up and get back to "normal," this family ended up doing a lot of self-sabotage and made things take much longer, which happens sometimes.

The therapist for the person who was victimized must ensure that the process causes no harm or distress for the client, even if that means inconveniencing other family members. Sometimes the victimized child can take a very long time before feeling comfortable with the idea of seeing the child who hurt them.

Sometimes it will not happen at all, which can cause a great deal of emotional and financial distress for the family. However, it is very important that the person who was victimized knows that they have as much control as possible over the situation and that their well-being is the factor that we are paying the most attention to. If the child who was victimized has a good relationship with their therapist, that can help control issues that may come up if the adults in the children's lives put pressure on anyone to make the reunification happen. Children concerned about angering or disappointing a parent can tell or demonstrate to their therapist that they are stressed, and the therapist can advocate for them. Sometimes not being able to reunify causes a great deal of stress for the adults and is problematic for the judge and others involved, as it can be difficult to find placement for a youth who cannot go home and does not have any other viable family options. However, the victim's well-being should not be compromised for the convenience of the other people involved.

Chapter 9

Treatment Content

Treatment for youth with sexual behavior problems often combines psychoeducation and more traditional psychotherapy. In other words, it is important for youth to have a place to talk about and process their thoughts and feelings about things going on in their lives, things they have experienced, and behavior patterns that are causing them problems. The space, time, and sense of safety needed to process their experiences are very important, and while treatment would not be successful without them, they are not the only things that are necessary. Youth also need to learn how their thoughts and feelings relate to their behavior, how to make healthy decisions, what is okay and what is not, and how to evaluate situations so they can use accurate information and healthy judgment.

As I said earlier, the therapeutic relationship is one of the most important pieces of a successful treatment program, but the program's content is also important. Not all treatment programs have the same goals or time frames, which will impact the content and determine which concepts get more emphasis than others. The individual needs of a specific client will also impact what content is necessary and gets emphasized the most.

Many programs use a treatment manual; there are a variety of treatment manuals on the market, and most of them are useful. Professionals must remember that the treatment manual is just the guide, not the treatment itself. The specific treatment manual used is often determined by several factors. Some programs are contracted to use specific manuals, and some manuals are better suited for certain populations. For example, there are ones explicitly written for younger clients or for clients with significant learning differences. Some treatment manuals follow a particular treatment theory, like the good lives model. Therapists might also choose a specific manual because it emphasizes certain concepts that are particularly necessary for an individual client.

I typically use a treatment manual called *Beacon*, written by my colleague Dr. Nicolas Carrasco, though depending on the client's specific needs, there are other manuals I use as well. Some clients are assigned to complete all the assignments in the treatment manual, some get assigned to do just some of the chapters that are most relevant to them, and some clients are assigned things that are not in the manual because they are relevant and useful for that child or are related to a specific issue that the court requested be addressed in treatment.

The remainder of this chapter will focus on some of the concepts typically part of treatment programs. It is not by any means a comprehensive list, and some programs will not include all the concepts, might have other concepts, or will spend more or less time focused on specific topics. Most of the examples and information in this chapter will come from the *Beacon* treatment book since it is the one I use the most. It is important to keep in mind that any specific program's goals, settings, and time constraints will greatly impact what information they work on teaching their clients. For example, more time-limited programs by design will have more narrow goals than programs with fewer time constraints.

Rules

By the time a person gets to the point in their lives when they are willing to inflict significant harm on another person, and often with sex crimes, the other person is someone they know and care about, there are usually a lot of layers of issues that need to be addressed. Clients have to process and deal with what they did, the harm they caused, and what was going on in their lives that contributed to getting them to the point where they chose to behave that way. Comprehensive treatment programs can take a great deal of time and effort for the clients and their families.

Rules, especially at the beginning of treatment, are an important concept to discuss. Youth typically have a number of probation and court rules their probation officer has given them to follow. In addition, treatment programs generally add lists of rules for the youth to follow while in treatment. While it does not usually feel that way to clients, probation is something of a gift. It is the court's way of saying that even though someone has done something that is against the law and has caused harm to others, the court believes that the individual has the capacity to prove that they can live safely in the community and follow the community norms and guidelines.

One way to show that a person can be a safe and responsible community member is to show a willingness and ability to follow the rules of the community they live in. It is also important that clients understand what rules are, how to figure out which rules they should be following, and what the purpose of the rules is.

Sometimes it is easy to figure out the rules because they are explicit and well spelled out. For example, the lists of rules clients are given by probation and treatment are typically written out and easy to refer back to. Some rules, however, are implicit; they are understood by people but often not explicitly spelled out. For example, I expect clients not to go through the things on my desk or rifle through my desk drawers, but it is not a rule I explicitly state to them when they are in my office. For most clients, it is an implicitly understood rule.

The definition of rules that I typically give to clients is that they are a set of guidelines that tell people what they should or should not do to stay safe and be responsible. Clients and their families need to know that while some rules are in place to protect others, many are there to protect the youth from the risk of being accused of something they did not do. For example, many years ago, a youth in our treatment program got into trouble at school when a teacher walked into an otherwise empty classroom to find him with his pants unzipped along with a few girls. When the adult came in, the girls reported that the young man had attempted to assault them while they were together in the classroom. The young man reported he hadn't, but since he was already on probation for a sexual crime, it was assumed he had. Luckily one of the girls fairly quickly came forward and admitted that she and her friends had actually cornered him and forcefully unzipped his pants without his consent, not the other way around. The young man was also able to take a polygraph exam to verify his version of events and did not get into any further legal or academic trouble. After that incident, we added a rule to the list that instructs youth not to be alone with classmates they don't know well to protect future clients from similar situations.

It is also important for treatment providers and probation officers to expect that clients will sometimes break the rules.

Suppose the client is in a treatment program or on probation with a county where the consequence for any infraction is severe and harsh. In that case, they are much less likely to be honest about their behavior and much less likely to talk about what is going on in their lives, and therefore less likely to get what they need from treatment. Clients who feel comfortable being honest about their behavior can get help for whatever challenges they might face before becoming a bigger problem. For example, a client who tells their provider that they have been struggling with viewing pornography again can get help figuring out what contributes to that behavior. Certain situations, thoughts, or feelings make it more difficult for them to avoid pornography. What is happening that is making the idea of watching appealing enough to outweigh the consequences? The client can work on figuring out what to do about the contributing factors to make pornography urges less frequent and more manageable.

On the other hand, if a client believes that by admitting they are struggling with pornography viewing, they will end up having significant and harsh consequences, and they are more likely to hide their pornography use. This will usually lead to more pornography use, as it may be difficult for them to figure out how to stop on their own, and also dishonesty in treatment will cause them to struggle with other aspects of treatment as well. When clients hide things from their treatment provider that they know they should talk about, they have difficulty making progress. It is very easy for folks to end up looking at pornographic images that combine sex and violence or humiliation, even if one does not set out to view those images in the first place, which can contribute to difficulties with a healthy sexuality and appropriate expectations in relationships.

Treatment programs, probation, and court systems must have reasonable expectations for clients and partner with them to help them figure out how to make healthy choices versus just a system for control and punishment. Of course, breaking some rules like "Do not touch others without consent" or "Do not be alone with children" may require more intervention than breaking a rule like "Do not stare at someone for more than two seconds." Community safety is the most important factor which needs to be balanced with the goal of clients learning how to manage their own behavior safely. After all, they will eventually graduate from treatment and be released from probation, and we want them to have their own internal skills to manage and not always need an external threat in order to function well in society.

Occasionally, I have worked with adult clients on probation in a county or with a particular officer who does not allow them to participate in any activities that have any risk at all, even if that risk is fairly small. This ends up in a situation where the client has had almost no chance to practice being safe in various situations while still having the support of therapy. This also often means that once the term of probation ends, the client goes from strict supervision and tight control to no supervision or external control at all without any chance to have a step-down period to give them time to adjust. Particularly for adult clients who have been on probation for a long time, the abrupt change can be overwhelming and difficult.

Risk

Learning to identify and manage risk is another important concept to understand well. Risk can mean different things in different contexts. For example, wearing a seat belt reduces the risk of physical harm while driving or riding in a car, and locking the car door reduces the risk that someone will take something that is in the car. For the purpose of treatment for sexual behavior problems, we are generally talking about the risk of getting into more legal trouble either by committing another offense or being accused of another offense. Clients must understand both types of risk so that they are aware that they not only need to manage their own risk of engaging in behavior that would cause harm to others and possibly get them locked up but also be aware that if they get accused of doing something sexual to another person without consent, it is unlikely they will be believed even if they are innocent given that they have a history of that behavior on record already. For example, we once had a young man in our program whose stepmother contacted his probation officer to report that he was having inappropriate conversations with his stepsister and making her uncomfortable. After some investigation, it became clear that those conversations never actually happened. It was not unusual for his stepmother to report him for bad behavior that he was not engaging in. It was important for him to realize that an area of risk for him was being around his stepmother. Not that he was at risk of doing anything to her, but being around her raised the risk of getting into trouble, even if he did not do anything. For most youth, being around their parent or stepparent does not raise their level of risk. Usually, it lowers it, but it was a significant problem for this adolescent. Unfortunately, avoiding his stepmother meant having less contact with his father, which was painful for him, but he could not risk going to jail simply because his stepmother did not like him.

Clients must learn to accurately assess the risk level they are taking in their day-to-day decisions. Some youth underestimate how much risk they are taking, which can create one kind of problem. Some youth overestimate how risky a situation is, which creates a different kind of problem for them. One useful way of assessing risk is to teach youth to identify risk factors for themselves and then see how those risk factors can combine to create a risky situation. Once clients can identify how much risk situations have, they can also identify ways to avoid or remove themselves from those situations if they need to or ways to minimize risk in the situation if that is the most appropriate response. Some things are risk factors for all clients, for example, being alone with a young child, looking at pornography, or feeling bored. Some things are specific to the individual client, like the example above of the young man whose stepmother was a risk factor for him, or perhaps a client who has realized that they tend to engage in problematic behavior whenever they feel lonely or ignored by a parent. It is also important for clients to identify where the risk comes from, whether it is something from inside themselves, thoughts or feelings, or something outside of themselves, like a person near them that they think is attractive. Knowing what increases the risk for themselves and where that risk comes from gives them a chance to figure out what they can do to minimize how often they find themselves in high-risk situations and how they can manage the level of risk they have when they are in riskier situations.

Thinking Errors

One of the most important and valuable topics for clients is thinking errors, more formally called cognitive distortions. Thinking errors are a way of thinking that allows us to avoid responsibility for something we have done or are thinking about doing. Using thinking errors makes people feel less guilty and more justified in their behavior. They are not unique to people with sexual behavior problems; pretty much everyone uses thinking errors sometimes, but for people who are engaging in inappropriate sexual behavior, they are usually the bridge between the idea of doing something that is problematic and actually engaging in the behavior. Thinking errors allow us to overcome or ignore things that normally stop us from engaging in bad behavior. For example, someone thinking about shoplifting might think stealing is wrong and consider the risk of getting caught, resulting in them deciding not to shoplift. However, they might also use thinking errors and convince themselves that it is not a big deal because they are only going to take something small, or are only going to do it once, or that it is okay because they are going to shoplift from a large corporation, or that they do not think they will get caught. The thinking error gives them the excuse that they can use to convince themselves that shoplifting is an okay thing to do. There are many types of thinking errors, and most treatment workbooks have a list of them for the clients to learn about. They all have in common that they are ways that we can make ourselves feel less guilty and avoid taking responsibility for something we are about to do or have done.

Some common thinking errors include:

- Assuming – this is when someone assumes that they know what someone else is thinking or feeling or how they will respond to something
- Poor me – this is when someone tries to manipulate a situation so that people view them as a victim or feel sorry for them.
- I can't attitude – this is when someone acts as if they can't do something when really they just don't want to.
- I forgot – this is when someone pretends they forgot something when really they just didn't want to do it.
- Anger/Let's fight – this is when someone uses anger to distract or intimidate to change the subject from something they don't want to talk about.
- Silent Power – this is when someone refuses to talk.

- Vagueness – this is when someone avoids being specific about something they are talking about in order to leave the other person confused or with the wrong impression.
- Minimizing – this is when someone tries to make something they did seem like not a big deal.
- Lack of empathy – this is when someone does not understand how someone else may be thinking or feeling.

I was talking to a young man who had just started treatment and was supposed to get a notebook or three-ring binder during the week between his appointments to keep track of his papers. He did not get it, which was unsurprising, and told me it was his parents' fault, which was a little surprising. He told me that he had written down on a note that he needed to get a binder and put the Post-it note on his treatment workbook. He did not, however, tell his parents that he needed a notebook. He also did not tell his parents that he had a post-it of things he needed sticking on his book or in any other way indicate to his parent that the Post-it note existed. He told me that he assumed his parents would know, go through his things, see the Post-it, and then get the notebook. In his quest to avoid taking responsibility for the fact that he either forgot or just did not feel like following through on what I had asked him to do, he used several thinking errors to avoid responsibility and any feelings of guilt about it and to try to convince me that him not having a notebook was the fault of his parents. Clients need to learn to identify and correct thinking errors when using them. I believe that one of the core values of treatment is to learn to be responsible, and without being able to understand and correct thinking errors, it is impossible to be responsible.

Positive Sexuality

Most people in the United States are uncomfortable talking about sex. Ironically, sex is used in almost all advertising and is common in movies, television shows, games, and music. However, it is not a topic that we tend to talk openly and honestly about. It is not unusual for adolescents who have gotten in trouble for their sexual behavior to decide, or sometimes be told by their treatment program or parents, that all sexual thoughts are bad. I once spoke to a treatment provider who worked in a program that required that their clients not masturbate at all, telling them that when they masturbated, they were creating another victim as the person they were fantasizing about did not consent to be in their fantasy. I believe this not only set the youth up to fail and encouraged them to lie, but it missed the opportunity to help them figure out what goes into healthy masturbation and healthy appropriate fantasies and what masturbatory practices are not healthy or safe.

When I work with adults who have committed sex crimes, I am often surprised by the lack of basic knowledge about how sex and reproduction work. Several years ago, I worked with an older gentleman with adult children and multiple grandchildren. Initially, he was resistant to looking at the positive sexuality chapter of his workbook, insisting that he knew all that. He was also quite sure that talking about it with his female therapist would not work for him. When we started going through the basic sex education information, he was surprised to learn how pregnancy happens and that a woman's menstrual cycle was involved. Even though he has had multiple children, he had never learned basic facts about reproduction. He had, all these years later, not understood the mechanics of how his wife had gotten pregnant over the years. He later told me he thought the information was interesting, and he was glad to know it, even if learning it involved what he felt were uncomfortable

119

conversations with the woman. I think it's important that treatment programs include information about the basics of puberty reproduction and other sexual information, along with information about healthy sexuality and healthy relationships.

Behavior Cycle

Another concept that is important in treatment is the offense or behavioral cycle. Versions of the cycle are used in treatment for many issues, including addiction. When clients are about to graduate, and I ask them what they found the most useful in treatment, they will tell me that it was the cycle. The details of the cycle will vary from program to program, but essentially it is a way for clients to see how events in their lives are connected to their thoughts and feelings and how that connects to their behavior.

Cycles can be created to examine the circumstances surrounding any negative behavior that might be useful to explore in treatment. Typically, in the treatment manual I use, we ask clients to create two cycles: one of some recent negative behavior that they remember quite well, like yelling at a parent or fighting with a friend, and then the second of their offensive behavior. These cycles allow clients to see any patterns in their thinking and feelings that contribute to them acting in ways that they later regret or get into trouble with. Once they can see those patterns, they are also able to notice when they are happening in the present and practice ways of stepping out of the cycle so that they do not keep repeating patterns they would rather stop.

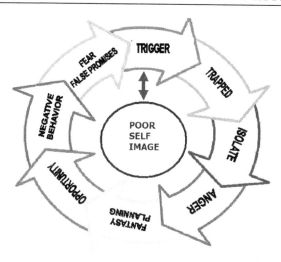

Cycle graphic included with permission:
The Beacon Therapist Guide by Nicolas Carrasco, Ph.D.

To create their cycle, clients first need to think about painful feelings from hurtful experiences that happened when they were very young. Clients are asked to list experiences that happened in their early lives and then list the uncomfortable feelings they had as a result of those experiences. We call that list of feelings the poor self-image (PSI). The PSI often contains feelings like fear, guilt, powerlessness, abuse, humiliation, rejection, and helplessness. For many clients, the list of PSI feelings can be very long. Since the PSI is established when a person is very young, it does not change no matter what behavior the cycle is about. In the image of the cycle, the PSI goes in the middle of the circle. Thinking about the painful events of their past and working on creating a list of hurtful feelings that they have experienced helps clients start to address and process the trauma that they have experienced, which is useful in their treatment.

Once clients know what their PSI is, they can start looking at the next steps of the cycle.

- **Trigger** - Luckily, people are not usually thinking about the harmful events or painful feelings that make up their PSI. Sometimes, however, something happens that reminds them or triggers them to start thinking about and feeling their PSI feelings.

- **Trapped** – This happens when the person starts feeling like there is nothing they can do to change or improve their situation or how they feel. They feel like they are trapped and stuck feeling awful.

- **Isolation** – People begin to isolate themselves, the next step in the cycle, feeling like nobody understands or can help. People can isolate themselves both by spending most of their time alone and when they are with others by not sharing their thoughts and feelings.

- **Anger** – The next step of the cycle is anger, when the isolated person finds themselves feeling angry at everything and everyone, usually including themselves.

- **Fantasy/Planning** – This is when people start thinking about what they might do to help deal with their anger. Usually, people have many thoughts and ideas, many of which get rejected as impractical or too problematic, some of which they may act on.

- **Opportunity** – This is when the individual finds or notices an opportunity to act on one of the plans from the previous step.

- **Negative Behavior** – This is when the person takes the opportunity to engage in negative or hurtful behavior. When working on the offense cycle, this is the step when the offense was committed.

- **Fear and False Promises** – This is when the person usually worries about the consequences of their behavior and promises themselves, or their victim, that it will never happen again. This leads right back to the Trigger step, and the cycle continues.

Once clients have their cycles written out, they can look at what feelings they had at each stage of the cycle and also what thinking errors they used to get from step to step. They can also plan what they can do in the future to stop themselves from moving through the cycle and deal with their PSI feelings and whatever trigger situations they encounter in a healthy and useful way.

Values

Discussions about values and how they relate to behavior can also be important in treatment. There are many ways to define the word "values." For treatment purposes, I usually define a value as an idea or belief that is important to me and helps guide my behavior. Everyone has prosocial and antisocial values, and some values, like power, can be either prosocial (healthy power) or antisocial (unhealthy power). Most of us do not sit down and list our values, especially the antisocial ones, and spend time thinking about how that impacts our behavior. Individuals who do this can see if the values they are acting out of are the ones they want to be most important and decide if they want to behave in ways that reflect the values they aspire to. For example, youth often tell me that education is an important value to them and their families. Sometimes that is reflected in the way they approach school, and sometimes it is not. Clients can also see how their personal values are the same or different from their families' values.

One of the young men I used to work with came from a family that valued power significantly. He noticed that in his family, especially for the men, that value was expressed through unhealthy power and violence. He decided to focus on healthy power and ended up being the first adult male in his family not to be incarcerated, a fact that he is very proud of. It took a lot of thought and self-reflection for him to figure out how to have the sense of power he wanted in his life without falling into the unhealthy patterns he saw in his relatives that he wanted to avoid. Figuring out what ideas and beliefs were important to him, what parts were the same, and what was different from his family was an essential part of his therapy journey.

Boundaries

Boundaries are also a fundamental concept to discuss in treatment. All clients in sex offense-specific treatment are there because they have violated a boundary. In the same way that rules can either be explicitly spelled out or implicitly understood, boundaries are sometimes quite obvious, like a door or a fence, and sometimes are implicit, like personal space.

Some boundaries are "place boundaries" and are related to location; for example, the area out of bounds in a sports game or the border separating two countries. Some boundaries are "people boundaries" and are related to personal and emotional space. All clients need to understand what boundaries are, recognize their own and other people's boundaries, and be willing to respect the boundaries of others.

Sexual Impulses

Of course, humans are sexual beings, and it is common and normal to have sexual impulses. Most people have hundreds a day without even really noticing most of them. Often, especially at the beginning of treatment, clients will insist that they have no sexual thoughts and never notice that their classmates or people they see in public are good-looking. While that can occasionally be true, especially for people who are very depressed, most people, especially teenage people, have sexual thoughts very frequently. Clients need to learn what is healthy and what is unhealthy. Once they can identify what is healthy and what is not, they also need to learn about what behavior is appropriate or inappropriate. For example, it is healthy and normal for teenagers to see a peer they find attractive and think they are cute. It might be appropriate to approach the person, introduce oneself and perhaps talk about the class assignment or something. But it would be inappropriate to think the person is cute and go up, kiss them, touch their body, or ask them to have sex. In this case, the sexual attraction (my classmate is cute) is fine. It is the fantasy that they have to be careful about so that they know if that is a behavior that is safe to engage in or not. Sometimes sexual attraction is not okay, for example, thinking sexually about a young child, a family member, an animal, or a nonsexual object. Those thoughts need to be stopped and redirected, as there is no sexual behavior that would be appropriate for anyone in those categories.

Different treatment programs break down the steps of a sexual impulse in different ways. Typically when I talk to clients about sexual impulses. I describe them as having five steps.

Five Steps to Break Down Sexual Impulse

1. Recognition
2. Sexual Attraction
3. Fantasy
4. Plan
5. Action

Step 1 – The **Recognition** step isn't necessarily sexual at all, and this is what happens when you see, hear, or are otherwise aware of another person around you. We automatically classify that person in our heads as being an adult or a child, and usually, what gender we perceive them to be as well. For people with sexual behavior problems, this is an important step to be aware of because recognizing that someone near them is a child is essential for following their rules and interrupting any sexual thoughts about someone who is not the appropriate age.

Step 2 – **Sexual Attraction** is when you notice something about the other person you like—for example, nice hair, cute outfit, nice legs, etc. At this step in the sexual impulse, I ask clients to decide if the sexual attraction is "normal" or "deviant." For treatment purposes, I define "deviant sexual attractions" as an attraction to a child, a family member, an animal, or a nonsexual object. If the attraction is to someone or something in those four categories, then the client must immediately stop the impulse. If not, then, so far, the impulse is fine.

Step 3 – **Fantasy** is when the person starts thinking about what they might like to do. For example, if someone sees an attractive person in the grocery store, they might want to look again, or if someone sees an attractive person in math class, they might want to ask for that person's phone number or if they can borrow a pencil. At this step, I ask clients to decide if the fantasy is appropriate or inappropriate. The fantasies described above would all be appropriate. However, if the person sees someone attractive and thinks about going over and touching them or asking someone they don't know if they want to have sex, that would be inappropriate. If the client's fantasy is appropriate, then it is okay to keep going with the impulse. If the fantasy is inappropriate, the client must stop the impulse.

Step 4 – In the **Plan** step of the impulse, people start thinking about how to make their fantasy happen. So if the fantasy is taking a second look at someone in the grocery store, they might plan to go back up the aisle they are in or just plan to turn their head. If the fantasy is talking to a classmate about homework, they might plan to leave the classroom at the same time as the other person so they will be near them to talk to them. In the planning step, I ask clients to consider whether their plan is safe or unsafe. In other words, if they plan to go near their classmate in order to ask their name or ask about homework, that is safe. However, if they plan to go over near their classmate, block the door, and back them into a corner so they can talk to them, that is not safe. Once a person decides if a plan is safe or unsafe, they know if they can move on to the action step.

Step 5 – **Action** is where the individual acts on the idea they had during the fantasy step. The action step should only happen if all the previous impulse steps are appropriate and safe.

A sexual impulse can sometimes happen very quickly and without much awareness from the person, for example, turning your head to get a second glance at a person you find attractive. Sometimes sexual impulses take longer and involve a lot more conscious thought. It is important for clients to start being able to notice and be aware of both the impulses that take more time and thought and the ones that happen quickly. That way, they are more able to make safe choices.

Honesty

Honesty is extremely important in treatment, and it is not particularly possible for a client to be successful without being able to be honest. There are a lot of things that get in the way of honesty for clients. Most obviously, clients often do not want to be truthful for fear of getting in more trouble. Clients also often lie because they are embarrassed or ashamed of their behavior or believe that the therapist or probation officer will be angry with them or judge them harshly. Sometimes youth are told by their parents not to talk about certain things or lie to their provider and probation officer about something going on at home. There are also times when youth lie about things to try to protect others from getting in trouble or being judged.

Honesty is emphasized throughout treatment, but we also have a chapter specifically focused on it. In that chapter, most of the assignments are about talking about what the client did during the offense they are in trouble for and having them explore what they were thinking, how they were feeling, and how they got past knowing that it wasn't a good thing to do. Some assignments ask the client to look at their whole sexual history, how and what they learned about sex from their family, friends, and school. What sexual things have they been exposed to, engaged in, or have been done to them? These things are not only important for the client to understand about him or herself but also important for the therapist to know so that we can be sure that the client is getting the type of treatment that is the most helpful for the individual issues that they have. There are lots of different types of sex crimes and lots of factors that contribute to any specific individual engaging in sexually harmful behavior. It is important to figure out what will be the most helpful for the individual client you are working with.

Learning New Skills

It can be difficult for youth and adults to know how to communicate their thoughts, feelings, needs, and wants to others. When people don't get their needs met in a healthy way, they often end up trying to meet those needs in unhealthy and sometimes harmful ways. When youth graduate from treatment, it is important that they feel more confident in their ability to get their needs met in healthy ways. One of the ways that I often discuss that with clients is to talk about the difference between passive, aggressive, and assertive. Youth can usually identify many examples of times when they felt like they let people walk all over them (passive) or when they responded to things aggressively. Typically for treatment purposes, I define assertive as the skill to confidently express your thoughts, feelings, or desires without hurting you or anyone else. It is more difficult than it sounds to express your feelings and thoughts to others, especially when you have had experiences with people reacting in unhealthy ways themselves. Learning to identify your own needs and communicate them to others is an important part of being able to function well as an adult.

Part of learning to express your feelings is being able to identify them. Youth also need to practice noticing and identifying the feelings that they have. Often, youth and adults have a fairly limited feeling word vocabulary, so they may sometimes be experiencing feelings and be unable to identify, let alone communicate, what is going on with them internally. It is important that youth in treatment be exposed to a large number of feeling words, know their definitions, and be able to start noticing when they, or others, are experiencing those feelings. It is also important that youth in treatment learn to take responsibility for their own feelings, especially anger. It is easy to blame someone else for making us mad (sad, scared, etc.). However, if our feelings are someone else's responsibility, then there is nothing we can do about it, and we are left at the mercy of other people's choices. If I am responsible for my own feelings and my reaction to them, then I get to decide how I will handle my day and be in control of myself. It is not always comfortable to take responsibility, but it is a lot more useful and gives the individual back their own power and control.

Empathy

Empathy can be defined as the ability to put yourself in someone else's shoes and understand what they might be thinking or feeling. Understanding how a victim of abuse may feel can help youth realize the depth of the harm they have caused and decrease the chance that they will do that again. It is much harder to hurt someone when you think of that person as someone with thoughts and feelings who might be in distress than it is if you do not understand or just ignore how your actions might hurt that person. Empathy is fairly easy to talk about but difficult to develop. Earlier I talked about helping youth expand their understanding of feeling words and their ability to notice those feelings in themselves. When learning about empathy, clients can build on that knowledge in order to start thinking about how victims of abuse, in general, might feel and specifically how the people they hurt might have felt.

In Chapter 8, we covered the clarification letter, which is one of the first steps in situations when a youth who has committed an offense is going to reunify with the person they caused harm. Typically, I have all clients write a clarification letter regardless of whether they will reunify or not because writing the letter is one way to focus on what the victim's experience might have been like. In addition, asking youth to notice and talk about times when others had empathy for them, how that felt, and when they have used empathy for others to help guide their own behavior can help them strengthen their empathy skills. As I mentioned at the beginning of this chapter, not all treatment programs will have exactly the same content and focus. Providers must keep up with the research in the field, so they know what is likely to be the most useful areas to focus on and, of course, individualize content to meet the needs of the specific client they are working with.

Chapter 10

Putting It All Together

This book is about working with youth with sexual behavior problems; however, you may have noticed that I have used stories about youth and adults with sexual behavior problems throughout the book. When the field of sex offense-specific treatment was emerging, providers made the mistake of taking the information they thought they knew about adults and applying it to children, which did not work well. I have found that the opposite often works. Much of what we know about successfully working with youth translates well to working with adults, adjusted for developmental levels.

I used to meet with an adult group in a more rural area of Texas. The individuals in that group could not come to my office, so we met in a room in the probation office in one of the local counties. One of the receptionists at the office once commented to me that whenever she walked by the room we were in, it sounded to her like I had a bunch of teenagers in the room with me. At the time, most of my clients in that group were at least middle age, but she was correct. It was not that much different from working with a group of adolescents, though, as far as I can remember, I rarely have had to address the importance of using deodorant in an adult group, and it can be a statement I need to make with some frequency in the middle school and high school groups. Besides body odor issues, one significant difference is that youths in treatment typically take much less time to progress in therapy and get what they need than adults, who have had much longer periods to establish and cement their behavior patterns and are more resistant to change.

Recently, a former adult client called me to talk about an experience he had at work. He noticed that he was able to handle his distress in a way that allowed him to manage the situation well and earn the respect of his bosses and co-workers. This person has spent most of his life believing that no one would defend or support him and that almost everyone is out to manipulate and control him. He is a former military member who was incarcerated for ten years due to his crime and then given an additional ten years of probation after his release from prison. When I met him shortly after his release from prison, he was very angry. He strongly felt that anyone in authority, particularly women, were not to be trusted and would be vindictive, volatile, manipulative, and out to get him. The first part of his time in therapy was not much fun for either of us. He was extremely unhappy, and he used most of his time trying every way he could to make me angry, so I would treat him badly and confirm his theory that I would mistreat him. He is a very intelligent guy, so the number of things he came up with to try and make me angry was wide, varied, and often pretty creative. Since then, he has repeatedly said that arguing with me was like trying to fight with water, which was his way of noticing that I typically do not power struggle with clients, even when they want me to. Even after several years, when he had finally decided I was probably not out to get him, it still was not unusual for him to get very angry, particularly if he felt emotionally vulnerable and try to pick a fight, and when that did not work, storm out of the room. He eventually made significant progress and was able to graduate successfully from treatment and complete the term of his probation. His difficulties in managing a relationship with me, his probation officer, and his fellow group members were replicated in relationships he had with family members, co-workers, and other members of his community, as he felt strongly that people would always be out to get him, and would be manipulative if given a chance. He is now more able to tolerate and manage his feelings when interacting with others or feeling vulnerable. This has resulted in him having genuine and respectful relationships with the people around him. He called to let me know that he realized his co-workers respected him and that he had noticed that, while he liked that, he found it so unexpected he was unsure how to handle it. This would not have happened without all the time he spent being treated respectfully by his probation officer, me, and his fellow group members. He needed a lot of that modeled to him. Since he was a middle-aged adult when he started treatment, the process took a long time. He likely would have moved through treatment much more quickly if he had been an angry teenager.

I wrote this book hoping it would be helpful, particularly for newer therapists in the field and for probation officers, judges, attorneys, and anyone else who makes decisions about treating and managing youth with sexual behavior problems. Sometimes we get siloed off into our own areas of knowledge, and we end up making decisions without some of the information that would be useful. While conferences and other gatherings can help spread knowledge, particularly in the age of the pandemic, it is not always logistically or financially feasible for people to attend every conference they might be interested in or benefit from.

Often, we can only participate in a fraction of the training we would like to attend.

This is a fascinating and fulfilling job, but it can be difficult to work in a job where the day-to-day decisions we make impact the health, well-being, and sometimes freedom of not only the people we are working with but others they come into contact with that we may not even know. We must take serious responsibility for our work and take care of ourselves, so we do not get overwhelmed or burnt out.

Nearly all the professionals I have had the privilege of working with over the years have been dedicated and invested, aware of the importance of treating the whole person, not just the behavior, and interacting with clients and their families in a way that reflects dignity, empathy, and respect. I hope our field will continue to move toward prevention and honor the humanity of all the people we work with, and remember that the quality of the therapeutic relationship is the most important factor for change.

Dedication & Acknowledgments

I do not think any book is possible without support and help from others, and this one was no exception.

In particular, I would like to thank Dr. Nicolas Carrasco, who was my supervisor when I entered the field and who I have worked with for more than twenty years. Much of what I know about working with youth with sexual behavior problems comes from him, and the information in this book is inextricably linked to his work.

David Walenta, LPC, LSOTP, polygraph examiner Sabino Martinez, and probation officer Lorena Moreno were all kind enough to read some or all of the book and give me their thoughts and feedback, which greatly improved the content.

Of course, none of this would be possible without the clients I have seen over the years. I am honored by their trust, courage, and willingness to do the work to live safe and responsible lives.

While I have been lucky enough to have good feedback and advice from my colleagues, all mistakes in this book are my own.

References

Adams, D., McKillop, N., Smallbone, S., and McGrath, A. 2020. "Developmental and Sexual Offense Onset Characteristics of Australian Indigenous and Non-Indigenous Male Youth Who Sexually Offend." *Sexual Abuse*, *32*(8), 958–985. https://doi.org/10.1177/1079063219871575

Caldwell, M. F. 2016. "Quantifying the Decline in Juvenile Sexual Recidivism Rates." *Psychology, Public Policy, and Law 22*(4): 414–426. https://doi.org/10.1037/law0000094

Caldwell, M. F. and Caldwell, B. M. 2022. "The Age of Redemption for Adolescents Who Were Adjudicated for Sexual Misconduct." *Psychology, Public Policy, and Law 28*(2): 167–178. https://doi.org/10.1037/law0000343

Harper, C. A. and Hicks, R. A. 2022. "The Effect of Attitudes towards Individuals with Sexual Convictions on Professional and Student Risk Judgments." *Sexual Abuse 34*(8): 1–25. https://doi.org/10.1177/10790632211070799

Harris, A. J., Walfield, S. M., Shields, R. T., and Letourneau, E. J. 2016. "Collateral Consequences of Juvenile Sex Offender Registration and Notification: Results from a Survey of Treatment Providers." *Sexual Abuse* 28(8): 770–790. https://doi.org/10.1177/1079063215574004

Harrison, J. S., and Eliot, R. S. 1999. "Polygraphing the Adolescent Sex Offender in the Residential Setting." *Polygraph,* 28(2), 176–181.

Laajasalo, T., Ellonen, N., Korkman, J., Pakkanen, T., and Aaltonen, O-P. 2020. "Low Recidivism Rates of Child Sex Offenders in a Finnish 7-Year Follow-Up." *Nordic Journal of Criminology* 21(1): 103–111. https://doi.org/10.1080/2578983x.2020.1730069

Letourneau, E. J., and Armstrong, K. S. 2008. "Recidivism Rates for Registered and Nonregistered Juvenile Sexual Offenders." *Sexual Abuse* 20(4): 393–408. https://doi.org/10.1177/1079063208324661

Letourneau, E. J., Bandyopadhyay, D., Sinha, D., and Armstrong, K. 2009. "Effects of Sex Offender Registration Policies on Juvenile Justice Decision Making." *Sexual Abuse* 21(2): 149–165. https://doi.org/10.1177/1079063208328678

Spice, A., Viljoen, J. L., Latzman, N. E., Scalora, M. J., and Ullman, D. 2013. "Risk and protective factors for recidivism among juveniles who have offended sexually". *Sexual Abuse* 25(4): 347–369. https://doi.org/10.1177/1079063212459086

About the Author

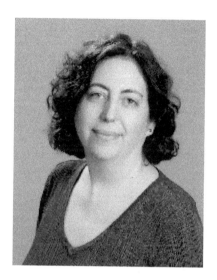

Shanti Duncan, Ph.D.

Dr. Shanti Duncan is a licensed professional counselor (LPC) and licensed sex offender treatment provider (LSOTP) in private practice in Central Texas. She has extensive experience working with people who have experienced trauma and with youth and adults with sexual behavior problems.

Dr. Duncan lives with her husband, two children, two dogs, two cats, and a tortoise. When not working or spending time with family, she enjoys gardening, reading, and playing music with others.

Shanti Duncan is available

for speaking engagements.

For details, please connect with her at:

12407 North Mopac Expwy Ste.250-285

Austin TX 78758-2475

shanti.duncan.lpc@gmail.com

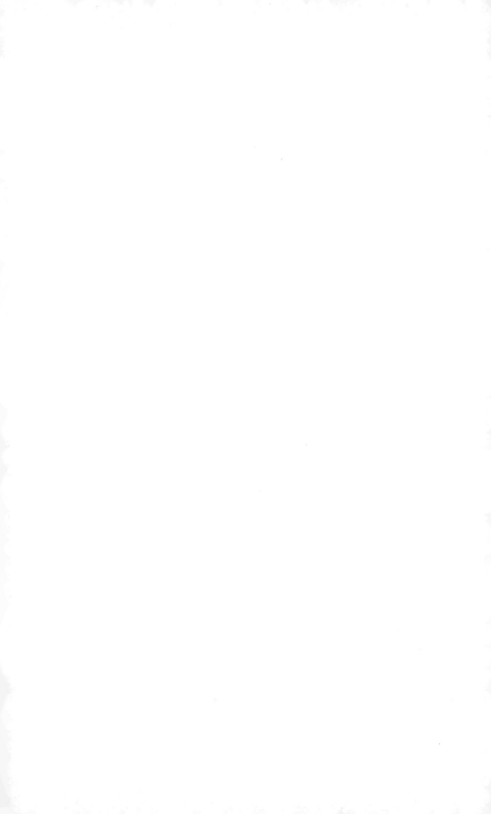